APPLYING QUALITY MANAGEMENT IN HEALTHCARE

A Systems Approach

Second Edition

APPLYING QUALITY MANAGEMENT IN HEALTHCARE

A Systems Approach

Second Edition

Diane L. Kelly

Health Administration Press, Chicago, Illinois
AUPHA Press, Washington, DC

AUPHA
HAP

Your board, staff, or clients may also benefit from this book's insight. For more information on quantity discounts, contact the Health Administration Press Marketing Manager at (312) 424-9470.

Library of Congress Cataloging-in-Publication Data
Kelly, Diane L.
     Applying quality management in healthcare : a systems approach / Diane L. Kelly. — 2nd ed.
          p. cm.
     Includes bibliographical references and index.
     ISBN-13: 978-1-56793-260-7
     1. Medical care—Quality control.   2. Health services administration.   3. Total quality management.   I. Title.

     RA399.A1K455 2006
     362.1068—dc22   2006043480

The paper used in this publication meets the minimum requirements of American National Standard for Information Sciences—Permanence of Paper for Printed Library Materials, ANSI Z39.48-1984. ∞™

Project manager: Jane Calayag; Acquisitions editor: Janet Davis; Cover design: Bob Rush

Health Administration Press
A division of the Foundation
   of the American College of
   Healthcare Executives
One North Franklin Street
Suite 1700
Chicago, IL 60606–3424
(312) 424-2800

Association of University Programs
   in Health Administration
2000 14th Street North
Suite 780
Arlington, VA 22201
(703) 894-0940

To Dan and Anna

BRIEF CONTENTS

DETAILED CONTENTS

FOREWORD

In the first edition of this book, I retold Don Berwick's story of how Phil Ershler, a world-class mountaineer, taught a group of climbers "how to walk and how to breathe" to illustrate my point that managers need to learn the difference between methods and results and that this book was about methods.

As the story goes, Berwick and a group of climbers met Phil Ershler, who has stood on the summits of Mount Everest and K2. Ershler was to guide Berwick and the group on their climb to Mount Rainier, which is no Everest but is a serious mountain nonetheless. Although Berwick had climbed Mount Rainier several times before, he arrived at the top exhausted each time. Now Ershler was the guide on his fourth climb. Before the climb, Ershler said he was first going to teach the group "how to walk and how to breathe." Berwick "thought he was crazy," and the group laughed, saying, "We are here to learn technique… not walking and breathing!" Six hours into the climb, Berwick and the group were no longer laughing, as "Phil had done exactly what he said."

According to Berwick, the habitual, unconscious actions of walking and breathing had been transformed into self-conscious, planned, placed, comprehended, and practiced tools for success on the mountain. The group learned the "rest step," the use of rhythms, the conservation of motion, the focus of attention, the alternatives in placement of the foot, and kicking and sliding at just the right time. The group studied equipment, the shape of snow, the position of hips and arms, and the optimal distances between members of the group. Walking and breathing, under Ershler's mentoring, had ceased being the simple, intuitive staggering and puffing of a neophyte with desperate eyes fixed on the summit. They had become a constellation of a dozen or more small and purposeful parts, each designed by experience, theory, and logic. Together, these learned parts added up to a new way, a transformation of methods. The next day of the climb, the group walked and breathed a new way. They arrived at their destination tested but fresh. Same mountain, new method, different experience. Berwick concluded his story with this: "Obsession with results is the impediment of improvement."

A lot has changed since the first edition, including the acceptance of evidence-based medicine and its extension to the broader area of evidence-based management, the expanding role of information systems, and the advent of various pay-for-performance programs as part of quality improvement initiatives. Yet much remains the same. Despite the growing acceptance of quality management, challenges remain to involving clinicians and managers in meaningful quality improvement methods that truly recognize the complexities of providing quality care. Thus, this book about how to walk and how to breathe within the complex world of healthcare remains as relevant and timely today as when it was initially published.

As with Berwick's mountain-climbing experience with Ershler, this book is not a comprehensive overview of various techniques but a systemic, integrated presentation of the fundamentals that managers need to know to make a difference in the practice of quality management. Each chapter is illustrated with relevant examples from the world of practice and is presented in an easy, readable manner. Exercises, along with companion readings, references, and relevant web resources, are included at the end of each chapter, providing the reader the opportunity to apply the concepts and methods discussed in the chapter. The chapters are presented in sequential form, building on fundamental concepts, underlying principles, and specific approaches for achieving quality results in complex systems.

However, the whole must be greater than the sum of its parts. Fulfilling this objective requires that the book provide an opportunity for the readers to synthesize the concepts, principles, and approaches. This opportunity can be found in the Epilog and in the Practice Exercise and Journal Exercise sections in which students can apply concepts to real situations and settings. The 2nd edition also recognizes that students and managers enter the learning process with different needs, experiences, and circumstances; thus, it offers readers different levels of learning. The book's focus is clearly on the learner, presenting real and timely lessons dedicated to methods of improving delivery.

As well described by Edward Deming, a pioneer in quality improvement, "the problems are with the system, and the system belongs to management." In this book, Diane Kelly has provided the opportunity for learning some methods that are analogous to Ershler's how-to-walk and how-to-breathe approach. These methods equip managers to address the problems and future challenges of the system for which they are the responsible agents.

Arnold D. Kaluzny, Ph.D.
Professor Emeritus of Health Policy and Administration,
School of Public Health, and
Senior Research Fellow, Cecil G. Sheps Center for Health Services Research
University of North Carolina at Chapel Hill

FOREWORD

The U.S. healthcare system has been through a series of "earthquakes" in its three centuries of existence. Perhaps one of the strongest tremors occurred in the early twentieth century with the publication of the Flexner report entitled "Medical Education in the United States and Canada." This report outlined the inadequacies of the medical education system and ushered in an era of setting scientific standards. It also marked the beginning of the construction of the world's most sophisticated, technologically advanced, and expensive healthcare system. Given these beginnings and Americans' support of technological breakthroughs, it is understandable that a common assumption exists that the American healthcare system delivers the highest quality of care. This perception persists, despite numerous scientific studies suggesting that the quality of care in the United States is highly variable and poorly measured.

As in other industries, public perception of the healthcare industry is often only altered by spectacular mishaps. Initially this view was driven by several tragic error-related deaths in the 1990s, which culminated with the Institute of Medicine's (IOM) report *To Err Is Human: Building a Safer Health System*. However, with new scientific studies suggesting that the healthcare system is not as safe or as effective as even the IOM report outlined, the demand for accountability has increased. More than six years after the IOM report was published, occurrences of tragic medical accidents continue, such as the clearly preventable deaths of a transplant patient at Duke University Hospital and a child at Children's Hospital Boston. These tragedies serve to maintain and enhance public attention to and concern about the quality of healthcare in the United States.

Predictably, these and other such events have energized politicians, regulatory agencies, and industry and consumer groups to focus on improving quality in healthcare, with ongoing proclamations, legislative and regulatory activities, and new reports on the subject. These activities in turn have energized the public to demand a much greater transparency for healthcare quality. As such, the Joint Commission on Accreditation of Healthcare Organizations is now requiring healthcare delivery organizations to track and report inpatient processes and outcome measures that are indicative of quality as well as to meet the ever-growing National Patient Safety Goals; much of this information is publicly released. In addition, other organizations have been formed to instantiate the public reporting of quality information; for example, the Hospital Quality Alliance has been created to coordinate public reporting of inpatient quality measures, and the Ambulatory Care Quality Alliance has been created to organize public reporting on outpatient quality measures. Perhaps the most important recent example is the success of the Institute for Healthcare Improvements 100,000 Lives Campaign—an initiative involving more than 3,000 hospitals that commit to implementing life-saving interventions and publicly reporting their results.

Clearly, a tipping point has been reached in providers' reporting of healthcare-quality results to the public. No longer will hospitals be able to use public-relations approaches to shape the public's view of the quality of care they provide. This information will now be controlled by other entities, creating a new era of accountability for the quality of care delivered by hospitals.

Although most healthcare delivery organizations can tell plenty of success stories surrounding their quality improvement efforts, many of these organizations have encountered barriers that have limited the impact of their quality efforts. These issues have included the cost of quality programs, the narrow impact of these programs, the inability to disseminate improvements throughout the organization, the difficulty of sustaining improvements, and the lack of true financial incentives in the marketplace for improved quality. Time and again, when these organizations get into financial difficulty, their quality programs are often the first to see reduction or elimination. Despite an increased focus on quality, many organizations are reeling from financial difficulties related to reimbursement issues, regulatory burdens, staffing shortages, and rising costs. It is fortuitous timing, as virtually all excess costs have been removed from most organizations through belt tightening; only a fundamental reappraisal of the processes of care (clinical processes in particular) can yield further significant savings while improving the quality of care. Nonetheless, without clear financial incentives, many provider organizations are hesitant to invest in new quality improvement programs.

The greatest healthcare earthquakes in the last half century have been related to changes in healthcare reimbursement. Starting with the introduction of Medicare in 1964 and followed 20 years later with the implementation of diagnosis-related groups (DRGs). Both of these tremors led to dramatic changes in the healthcare system. This will also be the case for healthcare quality as the U.S. healthcare system rapidly evolves from public reporting of quality information to using performance information to determine reimbursement. Several new initiatives have begun addressing the issue of paying for better performance in safety and quality of care, the best example of which is the CMS/Premier Hospital Demonstration Project, which has offered bonuses to hospitals that have the best performance on specific measures of quality. This program has made a dramatic impact on hospital quality performance, and significant cost savings have been cited. This program does not exist in isolation, as more than 150 different pay-for-performance programs now exist in the public and private sectors. Notable programs include the Leapfrog Group's Hospital Rewards Program, the Integrated Healthcare Association's Pay for Performance Program (in California), and the National Committee for Quality Assurance's Bridges to Excellence Program (in the Midwest and Eastern United States). All of these programs have begun to institutionalize the practice of better reimbursement for demonstrably higher quality of care. Although pay for performance has become a fact of healthcare organization life, its impact on reimbursement is only now being felt by hospitals. Yet the future is clear, and, like the implementation of DRGs 20 years ago, pay for performance's impact will be dramatic.

The second edition of Diane Kelly's book arrives at a critical point in this evolution. As healthcare managers increasingly see the impact of public demands for transparent accountability for quality, as regulators mandate the reporting of quality performance information, and as payers align reimbursement approaches to reward higher quality, managers will need to quickly develop not only a new skill set but also a core competency in managing quality. To date, expertise and critical skills in this area have resided within the quality improvement or quality assurance department and occasionally within clinical departments. Managing the quality of care has not been a critical skill for healthcare management nor an inherent part of the manager's educational experience. However, these skills are quickly becoming an indispensable part of any manager's knowledge base. Rather than long-winded educational programs that revolve around theories of quality, managers will need a practical guide to quality that is long on examples, adequate on theory, and easy to understand from the management perspective—a how-to guide for managing quality and safety. This is exactly what managers will get from this book.

Not only does this book supply the fundamental theory that underlies successful management of quality and safety, it also provides ample real-world examples and numerous exercises to help the reader quickly master the concepts. This book does not rehash old approaches in quality, but it picks up many of the fundamental issues and themes raised by the numerous IOM reports on quality as well as the latest developments in patient safety. It offers an integrated approach to quality and safety using a "systems approach" that overcomes many of the inherent limitations of quality improvement in years past. Organizations would do well to use this book as a principal educational tool for managers, and a required one at that. Indeed, this book will quickly become the manager's healthcare quality survival guide.

In the past, organizations focused on marketing the quality of care. In the future, this focus will shift to delivering quality and safe care as part and parcel of the business operations of any successful healthcare delivery organization. Organizations that do will thrive, and those that do not will see declining market share and shrinking reimbursement. Applying the principles and techniques in this new book is essential for any organization's continued existence.

David C. Classen, M.D., M.S.
Associate Professor of Medicine, University of Utah,
and Vice President, First Consulting Group,
Salt Lake City, Utah

PREFACE

Applying Quality Management in Healthcare: A Systems Approach is intended to help readers translate quality management theory and knowledge into practice. The book is easy to understand, and the real-life examples used to explain and illustrate technically complex concepts offer a highly leveraged approach to learning. The book does not provide comprehensive technical, medical, and policy background; instead, it explores managerial and organizational issues related to healthcare quality to assist managers who are or will be operating in various levels and types of healthcare organizations. The book is designed to enhance managers' literacy and awareness of concepts and practices that are required for effective management of health services organizations in today's changing environment. The goal of the book is to enable managers to work more collaboratively with quality experts who hold organizational titles such as chief quality officer, vice president of performance improvement, senior manager of quality improvement initiatives, director of quality and performance improvement, rather than to turn managers into quality experts themselves. While aspects of quality as they apply to healthcare services are discussed, equally important is the emphasis on improving the quality of the way health services organizations are managed.

Content Overview

The integrating theme of this book is systems thinking as it can be applied to healthcare organizations. Section I, "The Fundamentals of Quality Management," introduces concepts associated with quality management in healthcare and explains common tools for continuous quality improvement. Section I has been enhanced in the second edition to address stakeholder requirements such as those of the Leapfrog Group and the National Patient Safety Goals of the Joint Commission on Accreditation of Healthcare Organizations (JCAHO). Chapter 3 has been expanded to include two important patient safety tools: failure mode and effects analysis and root cause analysis.

Section II, "The Systems Approach," explores the influence of systems principles on quality management and introduces the concepts of systems thinking and dynamic complexity as expressed in healthcare organizations. In this section, several system models are presented to help organizations understand how relationships among variables within the system influence their overall quality results. James Reason's systems model for organizational accidents has been added to more specifically address system causes of medical errors. A new chapter (Chapter 6), "Expanding the Boundaries of the System: The Role of Policy," reviews the impact of the quality initiatives of the Centers for Medicare and Medicaid Services with a focus on public reporting of quality data and pay-for-performance initiatives; provides an overview of JCAHO's new accreditation approach, Shared Visions–New Pathways; and explains the basis for these initiatives and incorporates a systems approach to improving healthcare quality. The final chapter in Section II introduces the influences of systemic structure on sustainable improvement.

Section III, "Achieving Quality Results in Complex Systems," explores assumptions around common management activities and functions. Alternative ways of thinking about topics such as goals, measurement, and implementation are presented to enhance a manager's ability to achieve quality results. The Epilog synthesizes the information presented throughout the book. The Practice Exercises and Journal Exercise sections provide an opportunity for readers to apply these concepts to real situations and settings.

Because of the rapidly changing environment relative to quality in the health services industry, the structure of the text has been designed to remain current while the second edition is in print. Selected companion readings supplement the text with more in-depth technical content as well as extend the application of chapter concepts with relevant and current issues faced by healthcare managers and administrators. The companion readings and web resources in the text will provide readers with lists of leading authors and resources that may be further investigated for ongoing, up-to-date information.

The end-of-chapter exercises, Practice Exercises, Journal Exercise form, and web resources are also available on this book's companion website at ache.org/QualityManagement2.

The chapters are intended to be read in sequence, as concepts in each new chapter build on the foundation of the previous chapters' concepts. However, individual chapters may be used to present stand-alone concepts. The selection of topics, the sequence of presentation, and the types of exercises guide readers through the process of learning and practicing quality management.

Levels of Learning

The first edition of the text was composed of material developed for and taught at the University of North Carolina at Chapel Hill School of Public

Health in the Department of Health Policy and Administration. The concepts and exercises have been tested in the classroom and refined over seven semesters of teaching master's-level students. These students include those from the residential master's program and the executive master's program; those with limited work experience and extensive work experience; those enrolled in a variety of programs, including the master of healthcare administration, the master of public health, and the master in nursing administration; and those with nonclinical backgrounds. Physicians, nurses, respiratory therapists, occupational therapists, and nutritionists were also part of the test groups. The second edition builds on this foundation by incorporating feedback from those who have used the book as a primary text for master's students, doctoral-level students, and working professionals enrolled in continuing education programs in both in-person and distance-learning environments.

This book is appropriate for healthcare administration students and practicing healthcare managers. It offers readers different levels of learning according to their needs, experiences, and circumstances. The first level of learning is attained by simply reading the chapter content; this will provide an overview of the concepts illustrated through real-life examples. The second level can be reached by reading the chapters and completing the end-of-chapter exercises; this level is appropriate for a practicing manager. The minimum level of learning recommended for healthcare administration students can be achieved by reading the chapters and companion readings and completing the end-of-chapter exercises. The recommended companion readings supplement the chapters by presenting more technical concepts. Instructors may choose to assign any or all of the companion readings listed in each chapter.

The highest level of learning for both practicing managers and students is possible by completing the Journal Exercise for each reading and completing the Practice Exercises at the end of the book. The Journal Exercise is designed to allow readers to (1) reflect on the concepts presented in the chapter or reading, (2) practice formulating effective management questions, and (3) practice applying the concepts to real-world circumstances relevant to their own experience. Again, all the exercises in this book, as well as the web resources, may be accessed on the book's companion website at ache.org/QualityManagement2.

Acknowledgments

I extend my sincere gratitude to the individuals, students, teams, and organizations from whom and with whom I have learned over the years. Although it is impossible to list all of you by name, please know how important knowing you and working with you has been to the collective lessons presented in the book.

A special thanks to several colleagues who have influenced my thinking about the practice of quality management and systems thinking: Thomas Petzinger, Jr., David Tew, Dorothy Weber, Stan Pestotnik, Michael Goodman, Brent James, David Classen, Donna Fosbinder, Marj Peck, Harry Hertz, Steve Berman, and Jackie Mead. I also express my gratitude to colleagues who have been a source of support, encouragement, and collaboration: Elizabeth Hammond, Bill Shepley, Lynnae Napoli, Marla Birch, Joan Lelis, Karie Minaga-Miya, Robert Crawford, Patty Silver, Robert Silver, Marlyn Conti, Melissa Zito, and Terri Phillips.

A special thanks to the many students who have used and provided feedback about the first edition of the text. I would like to acknowledge Trina Bingham for her contribution to Chapter 3 and Daniel Nissman for his contribution to Chapter 8. Thanks, also, to the wonderful staff at Health Administration Press for their hard work, collaboration, and guidance.

I am grateful for the support from my academic colleagues at the University of North Carolina at Chapel Hill Public Health Leadership Program: Bill Sollecito, David Steffan, Willie Williamson, and Sue Havala-Hobbs; at the University of Utah College of Nursing: Maureen Keefe, Ginny Pepper, Emma Kurnat-Thoma, and Beth Cole; and at Weber State University: Ken Johnson. A special thanks to my friends and colleagues at Project HOPE and the many healthcare professionals in Lithuania, Latvia, Estonia, the Czech Republic, and Hungary, all of whom I am privileged to know. You have taught me that a passion for quality healthcare knows no boundaries.

Finally, I an indebted to my mentor, Dr. Arnold Kaluzny, whose continued support and belief in me made this book possible.

Diane L. Kelly, Dr.P.H, M.B.A, R.N.

THE FUNDAMENTALS OF QUALITY MANAGEMENT

CONCEPTS OF QUALITY MANAGEMENT

Objectives

- To introduce the concept of quality from a healthcare manager's perspective
- To define commonly used quality terms
- To define quality management as used in this book
- To describe a quality continuum for managers

A mother arrives at the pediatrician's office for her daughter's 6-month well-child checkup. As she has for previous checkups, she arrives ten minutes early and asks to occupy the well-child waiting area so her daughter will not pick up an infection from sick children in the regular waiting area. The scheduled appointment time of 10:00 a.m. passes, and so does 10:30, 11:00, and 11:30. The nurse politely tells the mother that the pediatrician has been called to an emergency, saying, "I'm sure you understand. If it was your child, you would want the doctor to attend to her." Although the mother understands the reason for the delay, this explanation really does not help the fact that she has to pick up her son from preschool at noon. The mother hunts for the harried nurse, who is grabbing a bite of her lunch each time she passes the nurse's station, to ask if her daughter may receive the required immunization shots and, if she could, to reschedule the rest of the checkup for another time.

Dissatisfied with the hours wasted at the pediatrician's office and disappointed with the need to return to finish the checkup, the mother demands to know if the pediatrician will be on emergency call during the time of the rescheduled appointment. When the mother and daughter arrive for the follow-up appointment, the mother hovers over the receptionist's desk so all of the staff will know she is ready and waiting. The office staff quickly identify this mother as a "problem."

Because the child received her immunization shots and well-child care in accordance with the guidelines of the American Academy of Pediatrics, one may conclude that she and her family were given high-quality medical care. Although the medical interventions were thorough and carried out according to the best clinical evidence available, the lack of quality management is what caused this family's unsatisfactory interaction with the healthcare system. In this example, the lack of quality management is illustrated by several circumstances: the pediatrician is assigned to both well-child

visits and emergencies on the same day, the patient-scheduling and queu-
ing systems are ineffective, and the office has a poor mechanism for communicating with patients and managing their expectations. These issues
have nothing to do with the quality of the medical care; they have everything to do with the quality of the patient's care.

This example illustrates important questions managers in health services organizations need to answer: What is quality? What is quality management? What is the manager's role in the quality process? This chapter
will begin to address these questions by defining management, describing
the relationship between management and quality, and clarifying common
concepts and defining terms typically associated with the word "quality"
and how it is used and perceived in healthcare.

Why Focus on Management?

Management, as it occurs within the context of health services organizations, is the focus of this book. With an increasing number of studies illus-
trating the gaps in healthcare quality in the United States (see Figure 1.1),
why is it important to focus on management? The reason is that all health
services are provided within and/or between *organizations*. Scott (1998,
10) refers to organizations as "social structures created by individuals to
support the collaborative pursuit of specified goals." A health services organization's methods of operation and specific organizational characteristics
may differ according to its purposes, focus, and values (Kelly 2002; Kaboolian
2000). However, whether the purpose of a health services organization is
care delivery, public health, education, or health promotion; whether the
focus of a health services organization is primary care, acute care, long-
term care, or insurance and reimbursement; and whether the operating
values of a health services organization are derived from an urban or rural,
a public or private, a not-for-profit or for profit, a sole proprietorship or
multifaceted institution, or an academic or community setting, all organizations need to do the following (Scott 1988, 10):

- Define and redefine objectives
- Induce participants to contribute services
- Control and coordinate these contributions
- Garner resources from the environment
- Dispense products or services
- Select, train, and replace participants
- Achieve working accommodation with the neighbors

While providing the actual service (e.g., perform cardiac surgery) and
producing the actual product (e.g., ensure clean water) are the functions of
the clinical and technical professionals, the organizational tasks listed above
are the functions of the various levels of management within the organiza-

FIGURE 1.1

Healthcare
Quality in the
United States:
A Snapshot

- In 2003, U.S. healthcare expenditures totaled $1.679 trillion and accounted for 15 percent of the gross domestic product (U.S. Census Bureau 2005; OECD 2005).

- In 2003, the United States spent more on healthcare, as measured by percentage of gross domestic product, than did any other country in the world; yet of 30 OECD countries, the United States ranked 22nd in male life expectancy at birth and 23rd in female life expectancy at birth, and 26th in infant mortality rate (OECD 2005; 2006).

- Fifty-five percent of those surveyed are dissatisfied with the quality of healthcare in the United States and 40 percent responded that in the past five years quality of care has gotten worse (Kaiser Family Foundation et al. 2004).

- Adult Americans received 54.9 percent of recommended preventive care, acute care, and chronic care (McGlynn et al. 2003).

- Between 44,000 and 98,000 deaths per year in the United States have been attributed to preventable medical errors, making medical errors the eighth leading cause of death—causing more deaths than motor vehicle accidents, breast cancer, or AIDS (Kohn, Corrigan, and Donaldson 1999).

- Taking into account direct costs (e.g., healthcare costs) and indirect costs (e.g., lost income, lost productivity, and disability), preventable medical errors cost the United States between $17 billion and $29 billion a year (Kohn, Corrigan, and Donaldson 1999).

- In 2003, more than 45 million Americans, or 15.6 percent of the 290 million U.S. residents at the time, had no health insurance (U.S. Census Bureau 2005).

- In the United States, persons between the ages of 45 and 64 years with the lowest levels of education have 2.5 times the mortality rates of those with the highest levels of education. Poverty accounts for 6 percent of the nation's mortality (McGinnis, Williams-Russo, and Knickman 2002).

tion. The scope, focus, perspective, and tactics may vary depending on the level of the managers (e.g., senior administrative, middle management, frontline supervisory); however, all persons serving in a management role or holding management responsibilities in an organization are charged with finding ways to accomplish the aforementioned organizational tasks.

Quality is not simply the responsibility of an organization's quality officer; patient safety is not simply the responsibility of the patient safety officer. Persons in these roles may be expert resources for helping managers understand; select; and implement tactics, interventions, and methods. However, the responsibility for ensuring quality and safe outcomes for patients, customers, stakeholders, and employees lies within those who determine how and what organizational objectives are set; how human, fiscal, material, and intellectual resources are secured, allocated, used, and preserved; and how activities in the organization are designed, carried out, coordinated, and improved.

The task of achieving quality outcomes from health services organizations is quickly becoming the shared responsibility of clinical professionals and management professionals. As Griffith and White (2005, 188) state, "just as medicine now follows guidelines for care; successful managers will use evidence and carefully developed processes to guide their decision making." The material presented in this book is intended to provide managers with evidence to assist them in improving their decision-making processes as they relate to quality and safety in their health services organizations.

Managers' Perception of Quality

The healthcare researcher's perspective may dominate definitions and approaches to quality in many settings. A widely accepted definition of quality, as given by the Institute of Medicine, is this: "The degree to which health services for individuals and populations increase the likelihood of desired health outcomes and are consistent with current professional knowledge" (Lohr 1990, 21).

How practicing managers in health services organizations define and approach quality in the context of their daily responsibilities, however, may be influenced more by their own background and experiences. For example, a physician assuming a quality management role may emphasize clinical outcomes and the implementation of evidence-based medicine or clinical practice guidelines. A statistician in that role may emphasize statistical process control and quantitative approaches. As a quality manager, a human resources professional may emphasize teamwork and team-based performance appraisal, and an epidemiologist may emphasize root cause analysis. A nurse in this role may emphasize a holistic approach to quality. Likewise, a nonclinical manager's educational focus can influence his or her preferred definition and approaches to quality. A manager educated in a business school may emphasize strategy, whereas someone trained as an accountant may emphasize the bottom line. A manager with a healthcare administration background may emphasize organizational relationships and structures, and a manager educated in public health may emphasize disease management programs.

These are just a few examples that illustrate the assortment of perspectives and preferences on quality in healthcare and the numerous ways it may be expressed within healthcare organizations. Given the multifaceted nature of quality, it poses several additional questions for healthcare managers: What is quality in healthcare? Which approach is best? How are the approaches related?

According to Dalrymple and Drew (2000, 697), "quality is conceptually complex and represents a synthesis of lessons, methods, and acquired knowledge from a range of disciplines." As a result, a healthcare manager can easily become overwhelmed by the complexity and extensive range of views on this topic. However, if the healthcare manager regards this array of perspectives as an asset rather than a barrier, he or she has the opportunity to draw from an expanded pool of quality lessons, methods, and knowledge.

As with management practices, the subject of quality in healthcare organizations has been the object of numerous trends, fads, and attempts at quick fixes. Because departments and professionals with "quality" responsibilities may change their job titles with the latest trend, managers must understand what is being done to promote quality in an organization in addition to how quality-related activities are being labeled. The first step for managers is to develop a common understanding of quality terminology.

Definitions

This section defines and clarifies the differences among medical quality, quality assurance, continuous quality improvement, total quality, and quality management.

Medical Quality

Since the early 1970s, Avedis Donabedian's work has influenced the prevailing medical paradigm on defining and measuring quality. In his early writings, Donabedian (1980) introduced the dual nature of medical quality by describing both the technical and the interpersonal components of care. He also identified three ways to measure quality—structure, process, and outcome—and the relationships among them. Donabedian (1980, 79, 81–83) described the measures in the following way:

> I have called the "process" of care...a set of activities that go on within and between practitioners and patients.... Elements of the process of care do not signify quality until their relationship to desirable health status has been established. By "structure" I mean the relatively stable characteristics of the providers of care, of the tools and resources they have at their disposal, and of the physical and organizational settings in which they work.... Structure, therefore, is relevant to quality in that it increases or decreases the probability of good performance.... I shall use "outcome" to mean a change in a patient's current and future health status that can be attributed to antecedent healthcare. The fundamental functional relationships among the three elements are shown schematically as follows: Structure ➡ Process ➡ Outcome.

For example, in an internal medicine practice with multiple physicians, the number and credentials of physicians, physician's assistants, nurses, and office staff are considered structure measures. The percentage of elderly patients who appropriately receive an influenza vaccine is considered a process measure, and the percentage of elderly patients who are diagnosed and treated for influenza is considered an outcome measure for this practice. The staff in the office (structure) would influence the ability of the practice to appropriately identify patients for whom the vaccine is indicated as well as to correctly administer the vaccine (process), which in turn would influence the number of patients developing influenza (outcome). Remember that process measures must have a demonstrated link to the outcomes if they are to be effective measures of quality.

Quality Assurance

A quality assurance (QA) approach involves eliminating defects. In an assembly line, defects refer to damages found in tangible products; in a service industry, like healthcare, defects refer to those performers who carry out a task or service poorly. For example, in a department that conducts insurance preauthorizations, several employees can accurately and speedily complete more preauthorizations than anyone else in the department. Alternatively, several employees, referred to as "dawdlers," can only consistently complete about half as many preauthorizations as the speedy employees. The rest of the employees are somewhere in between.

The department has certain productivity requirements or standards for the average number of preauthorizations completed per day per employee. The manager realizes that the dawdlers are dragging his productivity numbers down, so he sets a minimum daily productivity level for the entire department. After several unsuccessful attempts to meet the minimum productivity goals, the workers with the poorest productivity statistics are let go. With the dawdlers gone, the department's average number of preauthorizations per employee goes up.

Figure 1.2 illustrates this manager's QA approach. The bell-shaped curve on the left, which demonstrates a normal distribution, represents the combined productivity of all of the employees in the department; it shows the result of many employees carrying out the same process over and over. A measure of central tendency is shown by the vertical line in the middle of the curve and may be represented as a mean (average number of preauthorizations per employee), median, or mode. In addition, performance varies; a number of data points are at the "better" tail of the curve (the speedy employees), and a number of data points are at the "worse" tail of the curve (the dawdlers). The variation in employee outputs is represented by the width of the curve or the distance from the mean or average level of performance (the rest of the department).

The bell-shaped curve on the left may be thought of as the productivity before the dawdlers are let go. This manager's QA approach is to

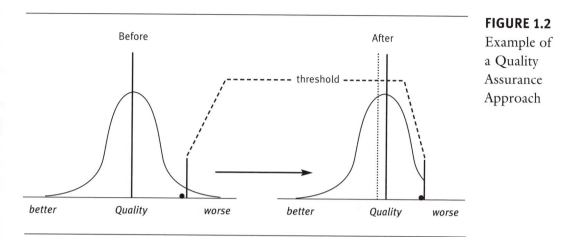

FIGURE 1.2

Example of a Quality Assurance Approach

Source: Reprinted with permission from James, B. 1989. *Quality Management for Healthcare Delivery*, 37. Chicago: The Health Research and Educational Trust of the American Hospital Association.

set a threshold of performance represented by the vertical line at the worse tail of the curve (i.e., the minimum daily number of preauthorizations per employee). This threshold causes the dawdlers to stand out. When the low performance of this group is formally identified and eliminated, the average number of preauthorizations per employee increases, which is represented by the dotted vertical line to the left of the mean in the bell-shaped curve on the right.

Quality Improvement

Faced with the same situation, the manager's interventions will be very different if he uses a quality improvement (QI) approach, which is also referred to as a continuous quality improvement (CQI) approach. The first question the manager would ask himself is, "Why are some employees really speedy and other employees take much longer to complete their work?" He talks to and observes the speedy employees first and the dawdlers next to understand how and why they take different amounts of time to do the same work. He asks the speedy people to get together, write down the steps they go through to complete a preauthorization, and offer any time-saving tips. The manager then calls a staff meeting so that all of the employees can learn how the speedy employees do their work. At the staff meeting, the department decides to adopt the speedy process as the new standard procedure. The speedy employees offer to train the rest of the employees in the department.

Figure 1.3 illustrates the manager's QI approach. As in the QA example, the baseline performance is represented by the bell-shaped curve on the left. However, the way in which the higher average level of performance is achieved is very different than what is seen in Figure 1.2. Improving the work process shifts the entire curve to the left, which in turn raises the

FIGURE 1.3
Example of
a Quality
Improvement
Approach

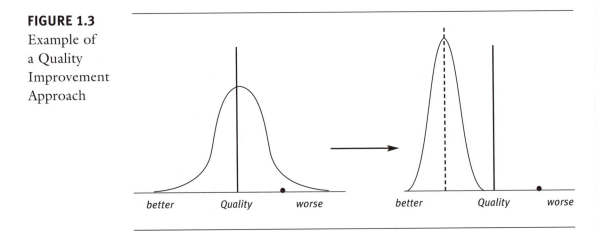

Source: Reprinted with permission from James, B. 1989. *Quality Management for Healthcare Delivery,* 37. Chicago: The Health Research and Educational Trust of the American Hospital Association.

average level of performance. By standardizing the process used to complete a preauthorization according to the speedy employees' best practice, all of the employees in the office improve their ability to complete the preauthorizations in a more timely manner. Although there are still employees who are faster or slower, the average time to complete a preauthorization improves. In addition, the distribution is much closer to the average, which is illustrated by the narrowing of the curve; there is much less discrepancy in employee productivity than before the change was instituted. In QI, the goal is not only to improve the average performance but also to reduce inappropriate variations in the process (James 1989; 1993). In this way, the process delivers the desired output or result on a more consistent basis.

Total Quality

Because the term "total quality" (TQ), also referred to as total quality management or TQM, is often used interchangeably with the terms "QI" and "CQI," students and managers may be easily confused by these two related but different concepts. The following definition clarifies the differences between TQ and CQI. Total quality is "a philosophy or an approach to management that can be characterized by its principles, practices, and techniques. Its three principles are customer focus, continuous improvement, and teamwork… each principle is implemented through a set of practices… the practices are, in turn, supported by a wide array of techniques (i.e., specific step-by-step methods intended to make the practices effective)" (Dean and Bowen 1994, 394).

From this definition, one can see that TQ and CQI are not the same; TQ is a strategic concept, whereas CQI is one of three principles that support a TQ strategy. Numerous practices and techniques are available for managers to use in implementing the principle of CQI on a tactical and an operational level.

Quality Management

Not only must managers understand the differences between TQ and CQI, they must also understand the differences between quality theory and management theory. Total quality "has evolved from a narrow focus on statistical process control to encompass a variety of technical and behavioral methods for improving organizational performance. Management theory is a multidisciplinary academic field... perhaps the fundamental difference between TQ and management theory is their audiences. Whereas TQ is aimed at managers, management theory is directed [at] researchers" (Dean and Bowen 1994, 396-97).

The overlap of these two schools of thought is referred to as "organizational effectiveness," a theoretical base that helps managers not only to improve the organization (total quality theory) but also to better understand and explain the organization (management theory) (Dean and Bowen 1994; Cole and Scott 2000).

In this book, the term "quality management" refers to the manager's role and contribution to organizational effectiveness. The book draws from management theory, quality theory as applied to non-healthcare organizations, and quality theory as applied to healthcare organizations to present practical lessons for managers and to integrate the unique characteristics of healthcare delivery and the context in which health services organizations operate. Quality management, for our purposes, refers to how managers operating in various types of health services organizations and settings understand, explain, and continuously improve their organizations to allow them to deliver quality and safe patient care, promote quality patient and organizational outcomes, and improve health in their communities.

Quality Continuum for Managers

Quality management does not just happen; rather, it may be viewed along a maturity continuum. Traditional or early attempts at quality represent one end of the continuum; mature approaches to quality represent the other end. The difference between early and mature approaches to quality in healthcare organizations may be illustrated by examining how hospitals prepare for a review by the Joint Commission on Accreditation of Healthcare Organizations (JCAHO). Following are illustrations of this point.

Hospital A is a large academic medical center. More than 12 years ago, its chief executive officer (CEO) demonstrated his support for quality by changing the QA department to the CQI department and hiring a director of CQI. Two employees, the JCAHO coordinator and the CQI coordinator, report to the CQI director. Three staff members report to the JCAHO coordinator; they are responsible for hospital accreditation preparation and for collecting and reporting the performance measures required by JCAHO. Five staff members report to the CQI coordinator; they assist teams throughout the hospital with improvement projects by providing facilitation, teaching improvement tools, and collecting and reporting data on the improvements.

Hospital A goes through a JCAHO review every three years, and the review preparation process has been the same for as long as anyone can remember. Nine months before the review, the JCAHO coordinator develops a master task list. The coordinator and/or his staff meet with every department manager to give out assignments and the timeline for completion. At the monthly hospital manager's meeting, the coordinator provides a progress report and announces the "countdown until Joint Commission." Three months before the review, the coordinator's staff works six days a week. The last month before the review, the CQI staff typically work 12 hours a day, six days a week. The level of stress in the organization gradually increases over the nine months of preparation, and the organization is in a state of frenzy a few weeks before the review. The surveyors arrive. The review is successfully completed, and the hospital even receives high praise for two of the CQI presentations the CQI coordinator prepared.

Hospital B is also a large academic medical center. Until ten years ago, the hospital approached the JCAHO review process in a manner similar to that of Hospital A. At that time, a new CEO was hired, and as she was getting acquainted with managers throughout the hospital, she asked a simple question: "What would happen if we operated every day as if the Joint Commission were coming?" Systematically, she began to create an organizational culture that she believed would be the answer to her question.

Hospital B also had two, separate quality-department groups: one group was focused on accreditation and one group was involved in facilitating CQI projects. The first thing the new CEO did was to merge the two groups into one and rename the department as the quality resources department. Rather than make the quality resources department the entity solely responsible for quality-related activities in the hospital, the CEO redefined the role of every manager throughout the hospital to include expectations for performance results, improvement projects, and JCAHO accreditation. Each manager was assigned a dedicated quality consultant from the quality resources department who would serve as a resource on measurement; data collection and analysis; JCAHO standards; and improvement tools, methods, and facilitation. Some quality consultants supported many small units, and some quality consultants supported a few large units.

The CEO also set new expectations for the administrators who reported to her. With her administrative team, she began to review monthly reports on patient satisfaction, financial performance, clinical outcomes, and productivity. As a group, they reviewed trends and discussed performance-related issues. After a year, the CEO asked the administrators to set their own performance goals based on opportunities identified from these monthly performance discussions. In turn, the administrators worked with the managers who reported to them to set department-level goals that were consistent with the administrative-level performance goals. All department managers were involved. For example, the pharmacy manager set the goal to improve the time to fill an outpatient prescription, and the finance manager set the goal to design financial reports that were more useful to managers.

The CEO also redesigned the hospital newsletter to include a "CEO Update" column that reported the hospital's performance and any business or market issues affecting the hospital. Finally, the CEO dug out employee satisfaction survey results from the past several years. She studied them as part of setting her own goals to address sources of employee dissatisfaction. She considered it her responsibility to create the culture and to provide the environment, resources, and tools that would best enable employees to deliver quality care to patients.

As the JCAHO review date approaches for Hospital B, announcements are made and final details are addressed. The week of the surveyors' visit is seen as "business as usual." The survey is successfully completed without much stress.

Hospital A exemplifies a traditional or less mature approach to quality. The focus is on meeting standards and eliminating defects. Quality is the job of specialists, while responsibilities for both JCAHO and continuous improvement belong to the CQI department. Progress along the continuum is seen when the hospital adopts CQI techniques to improve work processes. This point is demonstrated by the CQI projects sponsored by Hospital A's CQI department staff.

Hospital B exemplifies an organization that is progressing to a more mature state along the quality continuum. Hospital leaders demonstrate quality through their actions and through the direction they set for the organization. Quality is the responsibility of everyone in the organization rather than something that is delegated to specialists. Requirements of both internal and external customers and stakeholders are recognized and addressed. All processes in the organization—both clinical patient-care processes and internal operational and administrative processes—are targeted for improvement. Ongoing measurement and feedback promote an understanding of past and current performance to support the organization's ability to continually improve its results for patients and other stakeholders.

Although a healthcare organization may occupy a point anywhere along this maturity continuum, the goal of quality management is to continually strive toward the most mature end of the continuum. Figure 1.4 illustrates how the continuum may be viewed for healthcare organizations.

FIGURE 1.4
Quality
Continuum
for Healthcare
Managers

• Meet standards
• Eliminate defects
	• Products:
	  Healthcare
	  delivery
		• Products: All products,
		  goods, and services,
		  whether for sale or not—
		  care delivery, public
		  healthcare, payers,
		  equipment, supplies

	• Processes:
	  Clinical
	  procedures/
	  support
	  processes
		• Processes: All processes
		  —clinical, business,
		  operational, support,
		  manufacturing, decision
		  making, policy

	• Customers:
	  Patients,
	  physicians
	• Clients who buy
	  the products:
	  Patients, payers
		• Customers and other
		  stakeholders: Anyone who
		  has an expectation of, is
		  interested in, or is affected
		  by the work of the
		  organization—patients,
		  families, internal customers
		  employers, communities,
		  organizations, regulators

	• Cost of poor quality:
	  Financial
		• Costs of poor quality: All
		  costs that would disappear
		  if everything were perfect
		  —financial, quality of life,
		  productivity, opportunity
		  costs

Less Mature ——————————————————————▶ **More Mature**

Source: Adapted with the permission of The Free Press, a Division of Simon & Schuster Adult Publishing Group, from *Juran on Leadership for Quality: An Executive Handbook* by J. M. Juran (p. 48). Copyright © 1989 by Juran Institute, Inc. All rights reserved.

Conclusion

By understanding varied perspectives on how the term "quality" may be defined and the concept of the quality continuum in health services organizations, managers can begin to see

- how an organization can be successful at quality projects but not at attaining a quality organizational culture;
- why defining clinical practice guidelines does not in itself guarantee healthcare quality;
- why organizational development efforts, independent of clinical context, may not yield expected results; and
- why, without leadership's involvement in establishing a quality philosophy and strategy for the entire organization, only pockets of excellence may be found throughout an organization.

The rest of Section I provides a more in-depth discussion of TQ, beginning with the three principles of customer focus, continuous improvement, and teamwork in Chapter 2. The remainder of this book focuses on quality management by providing healthcare managers with practical lessons to help them in their journey along the quality continuum.

Companion Readings

Brook, R., H. E. McGlynn, and P. G. Shekell. 2000. "Defining and Measuring Quality of Care: A Perspective from US Researchers." *International Journal for Quality in Healthcare* 12 (4): 281–95.

Centers for Disease Control and Prevention. *Health, United States, with Chartbook on Trends in the Health of Americans.* Hyattsville, MD: National Center for Health Statistics. (See especially the Executive Summary and Highlights).

Griffith, J. R., and K. R. White. 2005. "The Revolution in Hospital Management." *Journal of Healthcare Management* 50 (3): 170–90.

Web Resources

Institute of Medicine Quality Initiative. The following publications are available on www.iom.edu:
- To Err Is Human: Building a Safer Health System
- Crossing the Quality Chasm: A New Health System for the 21st Century
- Envisioning the National Health Care Quality Report
- Keeping Patient's Safe: Transforming the Work Environment of Nurses
- Quality Through Collaboration: The Future of Rural Health

Agency for Healthcare Research and Quality. The following publications are available on www.qualitytools.ahrq.gov/:
- The National Healthcare Quality Report
- The National Healthcare Disparities Report

Centers for Disease Control and Prevention, National Center for Health Statistics. This is available on www.cdc.gov/nchs/hus.htm:
- *Health, United States*

U.S. Census Bureau. This is available on www.census.gov/statab/www:
- *Statistical Abstract of the United States, 2006 Edition*

References

Cole, R. E., and W. R. Scott (eds.). 2000. *The Quality Movement and Organization Theory.* Thousand Oaks, CA: Sage Publications.

Dalrymple, J., and E. Drew. 2000. "Quality: On the Threshold or the Brink?" *Total Quality Management* 11 (4–6): 697–703.

Dean, J. W., and D. E. Bowen. 1994. "Management Theory and Total Quality: Improving Research and Practice Through Theory Development." *Academy of Management Review* 19 (2): 392–418.

Donabedian, A. 1980. *Explorations in Quality Assessment and Monitoring, Volume 1: The Definition of Quality and Approaches to Its Assessment.* Chicago: Health Administration Press.

Griffith, J. R., and K. R. White. 2005. "The Revolution in Hospital Management." *Journal of Healthcare Management* 50 (3): 170–90.

James, B. 1989. *Quality Management for Healthcare Delivery.* Chicago: The Health Research and Educational Trust of the American Hospital Association.

———. 1993. "Implementing Practice Guidelines Through Clinical Quality Improvement." *Frontiers of Health Services Management* 10 (1): 3–37.

Juran, J. M. 1989. *Juran on Leadership for Quality: An Executive Handbook.* New York: The Free Press.

Kaboolian, L. 2000. "Quality Comes to the Public Sector." In *The Quality Movement and Organizational Theory*, edited by R. E. Core and W. R. Scott, 131-53. Thousand Oaks, CA: Sage Publications.

Kaiser Family Foundation, Agency for Healthcare Research and Quality, and Harvard School of Public Health. 2004. *National Survey on Consumers' Experiences with Patient Safety and Quality Information.* Menlo Park, CA: Kaiser Family Foundation.

Kelly, D. L. 2002. "Using the Baldrige Criteria for Improving Performance in Public Health." Ph.D. dissertation, University of North Carolina at Chapel Hill.

Kohn, L. T., J. M. Corrigan, and M. S. Donaldson (eds.), Committee on Quality of Healthcare in America, Institute of Medicine. 1999. *To Err Is Human: Building a Safer Health System.* Washington, DC: National Academies Press.

Lohr, K. N. (ed.). 1990. *Medicare: A Strategy for Quality Assurance.* Washington, DC: National Academies Press.

McGinnis, J. M., P. Williams-Russo, and J. R. Knickman. 2002. "The Case for More Active Policy Attention to Promotion." *Health Affairs* 21 (2): 78–93.

McGlynn, E. A., S. M. Asch, J. Adams, J. Keesy, J. Hicks, A. DeCristofaro, and E. A. Kerr. 2003. "The Quality of Health Care Delivered to Adults in the United States." *New England Journal of Medicine* 348 (26): 2635–45.

Organisation for Economic Co-operation and Development (OECD). 2006. *OECD Factbook, 2006: Economic, Environmental and Social Statistics.* [Online information; retrieved 5/4/06.] www.oecd.org/document/62 /0,2340,en_21571361_34374092_34420734_1_1_1_1,00.html.

———. 2005. *OECD Health Data 2005: Statistics and Indicators for 30 Countries.* [Online information; retrieved 5/4/06.] www.oecd.org /document/30/0,2340,en_2825_495642_12968734_1_1_1_1,00.html.

Scott, R. A. 1998. *Organizations: Rational, Natural, and Open Systems, 4th Edition.* Upper Saddle River, NJ: Prentice Hall.

U.S. Census Bureau. 2005. *Statistical Abstract of the United States, 2004–2005.* [Online information; retrieved 10/24/05.] www.census.gov/statab /www/vital.html.

Exercise

This exercise may also be accessed on this book's companion website at ache.org/QualityManagement2.

Objective: To explore how managers influence the quality of products, services, and the customer experience.

Instructions:

1. Think of an experience where you received or observed excellent quality. You may have had this experience as a customer, as a patient, as a provider, or as an employee. Describe the factors that made this an excellent experience and how you felt as a result of this experience. Using the list of management functions listed in this chapter as a guide, include a description of management's influence on your experience. Do the same for a situation in which you experienced poor quality. Record your responses in the table below or on one similar to it.

	Briefly describe the experience.	Describe what made this an excellent or poor quality experience.	How did you feel as a result?	What was management's role or influence?
Excellent Quality				
Poor Quality				

2. On the basis of the observations you recorded in the table, describe why it is important for healthcare managers to understand quality.

THREE PRINCIPLES OF TOTAL QUALITY

Objectives

- To describe the three principles of total quality: customer focus, continuous improvement, and teamwork
- To begin to explore how these three principles may be expressed in the managerial role
- To practice identifying management behaviors that demonstrate these three principles

Any healthcare manager would probably say that quality patient care, quality outcomes, or health improvement factored into their decision to pursue a career in healthcare. However, translating a commitment to quality into management actions and interactions has remained elusive to managers. The previous chapter defined total quality as "a philosophy or an approach to management that can be characterized by its principles, practices, and techniques. Its three principles are customer focus, continuous improvement, and teamwork" (Dean and Bowen 1994, 394). In this chapter, you will begin to explore how managers may strategically integrate the principles of TQ into how they carry out managerial functions.

The information presented in this chapter is not intended to replace management knowledge and skills in areas such as finance, human resources, strategy, or marketing; rather, this information should complement those areas. By viewing their role through a TQ lens, managers may enhance their overall ability to use their range of knowledge. By doing this, they will be better able to achieve desired results within their scope of responsibility, whether for an entire organization, a department, or a team.

Principle 1: Customer Focus

The principle of customer focus may be better applied when the manager is aware of the dual nature of medical quality and is able to define customers and stakeholders as well as their respective expectations and requirements.

Dual Nature of Quality

Managers must remember that many clinical healthcare professionals have been educated in a philosophy that defines quality according to the professional's expertise and expectations rather than according to the patient's, customer's, and stakeholder's expectations or requirements. In Chapter 1, the dual nature of medical quality, as described by Donabedian (technical and interpersonal components of care), was introduced. The term "content quality" refers to clinical expertise and technical aspects of healthcare (e.g., selecting the appropriate intervention for a patient's symptoms or carrying out a clinical procedure properly). Most patients assume that providers possess and deliver technical quality. The terms "delivery quality" and "service quality" refer to the interpersonal components of care (e.g., empathy and communication) and to how well a patient's requirements and expectations are being met (e.g., access, timely billing) (James 1989).

To manage from a TQ philosophy, managers should first determine the extent to which they themselves, as well as providers and other employees, understand and accept the dual nature of quality. Managers, as departmental or organizational leaders, are responsible for establishing a customer-focused environment and direction for their employees. This comment from a skilled technical nurse—"I wish the family would get out of the way so I could do my job"—suggests a work environment in which content quality is valued and rewarded above service quality. Policies and procedures, job descriptions, personnel performance expectations and evaluations, reward systems, and staff development may be viewed as tools to help managers create a customer-focused environment. By purposefully and strategically incorporating both aspects of quality care into the design of these management tools, managers may enhance their ability to implement a focus on both content quality and service quality.

Beyond Service Quality: Meeting Customer and Stakeholder Requirements

A customer is anyone who has an expectation about the output of a process (James 1989). External customers are the parties outside the organization, and the primary external customers for healthcare providers are patients, families, and significant others. The customer-focus principle requires managers who are operating from a TQ philosophy to be attentive not only to their external customers but also to their internal customers and stakeholders. An internal customer comes from within the organization. This type of customer may be someone who is responsible for activities that are "downstream" from the ones somebody else is doing. For example, in a hospital, when patient care is handed off from one provider to another at shift change, the incoming provider is considered the internal customer of the outgoing provider. Completing the requisite shift responsibilities in a timely manner, communicating relevant information, and leaving a tidy work space demonstrate recognition of coworkers as internal customers.

In the past, quality management defined the customer as the user of the products or services (i.e., process outputs). The contemporary view of quality management expands the concept of "customer" to include stakeholders and markets in which the organization operates. The term "stakeholder" is used to refer to "all groups that are or might be affected by an organization's services, actions or success" (National Institute for Standards and Technology 2006, 75). In healthcare organizations, stakeholders may include "insurers and other third party payors, employers, health care providers, patient advocacy groups, Departments of Health, staff, partners, governing boards, investors, charitable contributors, suppliers, taxpayers, policymakers, and local and professional communities" (National Institutes for Standards and Technology 2006, 75). Defining customers and stakeholders is a prerequisite to determining their requirements and, in turn, to designing organizational processes that meet these requirements.

In addition to behaviors at the interpersonal level (such as courtesy), operating from a customer-focused position requires an understanding not only of who the customers are but also of what these customers require; how the requirements differ between customer groups; how these requirements change over time; and how these requirements guide organizational strategy, decisions, and activities (National Institutes for Standards and Technology 2006). Patients as customer groups may be differentiated by disease category (e.g., cancer, cardiovascular, obstetrics), age, the nature of the illness (e.g., chronic, acute), the site of care (e.g., inpatient, outpatient, long-term care), ethnicity, or language. The advent of evening outpatient clinic hours illustrates how organizational decisions on hours of operation have changed to keep pace with changing patient work schedules and employment requirements. Adopting culturally competent approaches to patient care, incorporating translation services, and providing patient education materials in multiple languages are examples of how organizations have adapted their internal operations to meet the needs of ethnically diverse communities.

Stakeholders' Quality Requirements

In recent years, regulatory and payer stakeholders have assumed increasingly influential roles in promoting the quality agenda in healthcare. Since 1996, JCAHO has taken a more prescriptive stand on patient safety in the accreditation process. In 1996, JCAHO implemented its sentinel event policy; in 2001, JCAHO added standards describing the organizational leadership's role in patient safety; and in 2003, JCAHO incorporated the first, formalized set of safety requirements for direct patient-care activities (see www.jcaho.org; Devers, Pham, and Liu 2004). These requirements, based on studies of safe practices, are called the National Patient Safety Goals (NPSGs) and have evolved to include nine settings of care, including hospitals, home care, ambulatory surgery, and laboratories. Table 2.1 shows the 2004 and 2006 NPSGs for hospitals to illustrate the changing nature of these key stakeholder requirements. The NPSGs have implications for

TABLE 2.1
JCAHO's
National
Patient Safety
Goals:
Changes from
2004 to 2006

2004	2006
Improve the accuracy of patient identification. • Use at least two patient identifiers (neither to be the patient's room number) whenever taking blood samples or administering medications or blood products. • Prior to the start of any surgical or invasive procedure, conduct a final verification process, such as a "time out," to confirm the correct patient, procedure, and site, using active—not passive—communication techniques. **Improve the effectiveness of communication among caregivers.** • Implement a process for taking verbal or telephone orders or critical test results that require a verification "read back" of the complete order or test result by the person receiving the order or test result. • Standardize the abbreviations, acronyms, and symbols used throughout the organization, including a list of abbreviations, acronyms, and symbols not to use. **Improve the safety of using high-alert medications.** • Remove concentrated electrolytes (including, but not limited to, potassium chloride, potassium phosphate, sodium chloride >0.9%) from patient care units. • Standardize and limit the number of drug concentrations available in the organization.	**Improve the accuracy of patient identification.** • Use at least two patient identifiers (neither to be the patient's room number) whenever taking blood samples, or administering medications or blood products and other specimens for clinical testing, or providing any other treatments or procedures. **Improve the effectiveness of communication among caregivers.** • Implement a process for taking verbal or telephone orders or critical test results that require a verification "read-back" of the complete order or test result by the person receiving the order or test result. • Standardize the abbreviations, acronyms, and symbols used throughout the organization, including a list of abbreviations, acronyms, and symbols not to use. • Measure, assess, and, if appropriate, take action to improve the timeliness of reporting and the timeliness of receipt by the responsible licensed caregiver, of critical test results and values. • Implement a standardized approach to "hand off" communications, including an opportunity to ask and respond to questions. **Improve the safety of using medications.** • Standardize and limit the number of drug concentrations available in the organization. • Identify and, at a minimum, annually review a list of look-alike/sound-alike drugs used in the organization, and take action to prevent errors involving the interchange of these drugs. • Label all medications, medication containers (e.g., syringes, medicine cups, basins), or other solutions on and off the sterile field in perioperative and other procedural settings.

continued

2004	2006	TABLE 2.1 *(Continued)*

2004	2006
Eliminate wrong-site, wrong-patient, wrong-procedure surgery. • Create and use a preoperative verification process, such as a checklist, to confirm that appropriate documents (e.g., medical records, imaging studies) are available. • Implement a process to mark the surgical site and involve the patient in the marking process.	**Reduce the risk of health care-acquired infections.** • Comply with current CDC hand hygiene guidelines. • Manage as sentinel events all identified cases of unanticipated death or major permanent loss of function associated with a health care-acquired infection.
Improve the safety of using infusion pumps. • Ensure free-flow protection on all general-use and PCA (patient-controlled analgesia) intravenous infusion pumps used in the organization.	**Accurately and completely reconcile medications across the continuum of care.** • Develop a process for obtaining and documenting a complete list of the patient's current medications upon the patient's admission to the organization and with the involvement of the patient. This process includes a comparison of the medications the organization provides to those on the list.
Improve the effectiveness of clinical alarm systems. • Implement regular preventive maintenance and testing of alarm systems. • Assure that alarms are activated with appropriate settings and are sufficiently audible with respect to distances and competing noise within the unit.	• A complete list of the patient's medications is communicated to the next provider of service when it refers or transfers a patient to another setting, service, practitioner, or level of care within or outside the organization.
Reduce the risk of health care-acquired infections. • Comply with current CDC hand hygiene guidelines. • Manage as sentinel events all identified cases of unanticipated death or major permanent loss of function associated with a health care-acquired infection.	**Reduce the risk of patient harm resulting from falls.** • Implement a fall reduction program and evaluate the effectiveness of the program.

Source: © Joint Commission on Accreditation of Healthcare Organizations, 2004, 2006. Reprinted with permission.

how managers make decisions about capital equipment (i.e., infusion pumps), preventive maintenance (i.e., patient monitors), procurement (i.e., pharmaceuticals), and training (i.e., Centers for Disease Control and Prevention [CDC] hand-washing guidelines). The NPSGs have implications for how managers prioritize improvements (i.e., fall-reduction program), establish communication systems between departments (i.e., laboratory staff and care providers), establish communication between sites of care (i.e., medication reconciliation), and evaluate documentation tools (i.e., "do not use" abbreviations) (JCAHO 2005).

The role of payers as stakeholders in the quality agenda has also evolved in recent years. In addition to insurance companies and government programs, such as Medicare, employers who provide health insurance as an employee benefit must also be considered as "payers." The Leapfrog Group is one of the most influential of this new type of stakeholder. The Leapfrog Group is a "growing consortium of Fortune 500 companies and other large private and public healthcare purchasers that provide health benefits to more than 34 million Americans in all 50 states... and... spend tens of billions of dollars on health care annually. Leapfrog members have agreed to base their purchase of health care on principles that encourage provider quality improvement and consumer involvement" (The Leapfrog Group 2005).

Leapfrog members have endorsed specific safe practices as negotiating points between employers and health plans. Figure 2.1 summarizes those practices as well as the principles guiding employer health plan purchases. While initially targeting hospitals, the Leapfrog Group's requirements are not insignificant for managers in the areas of capital planning and investment (e.g., computerized physician order entry), human resources management and physician relations (e.g., intensivists), service mix and revenue sources (e.g., evidence-based hospital referral), and operational transparency (e.g., Leapfrog safe practices score).

Federal and state governments are additional examples of stakeholders whose requirements for health services organizations are changing and evolving, particularly in the areas of quality reporting. The topics of "transparency" and quality reporting are discussed in more detail in chapters 6 and 10.

Principle 2: Continuous Improvement

The principle of continuous improvement may be expressed through managers' day-to-day actions and how they execute their managerial functions.

Day-to-Day Actions

It is not uncommon for the manager of an environmental services department in a large hospital to pick up something from the hallway floor and

FIGURE 2.1

The Leapfrog Group's Safe Practices

The Leapfrog Group identified and has since refined four hospital quality and safety practices that are the focus of its health care provider performance comparisons and hospital recognition and reward. Based on independent scientific evidence, the quality practices are: computer physician order entry; evidence-based hospital referral; intensive care unit (ICU) staffing by physicians experienced in critical care medicine; and The Leapfrog Safe Practices Score, based on the NQF-endorsed safe practices.

- Computer Physician Order Entry (CPOE): With CPOE systems, hospital staff enter medication orders via computers linked to prescribing error-prevention software. CPOE has been shown to reduce serious prescribing errors in hospitals by more than 50%.
- Evidence-based Hospital Referral (EHR): Consumers and health care purchasers should choose hospitals with extensive experience and the best results with certain high-risk surgeries and conditions. By referring patients needing certain complex medical procedures to hospitals offering the best survival odds based on scientifically valid criteria—such as the number of times a hospital performs these procedures each year or other process or outcomes data—research indicates that a patient's risk of dying could be reduced by 40%.
- ICU Physician Staffing (IPS): Staffing ICUs with doctors who have special training in critical care medicine, called "intensivists," has been shown to reduce the risk of patients dying in the ICU by 40%.
- The Leapfrog Safe Practices Score–the National Quality Forum's 27 Safe Practices: The National Quality Forum-endorsed 30 Safe Practices cover a range of practices that, if utilized, would reduce the risk of harm in certain processes, systems, or environments of care. Included in the 30 practices are the original 3 Leapfrog leaps. For this new leap, added in April 2004, hospitals' progress on the remaining 27 safe practices will be assessed.

This list is based on four primary criteria:
1. There is overwhelming scientific evidence that these quality and safety leaps will significantly reduce preventable medical mistakes.
2. Their implementation by the health industry is feasible in the near term.
3. Consumers can readily appreciate their value.
4. Health plans, purchasers, or consumers can easily ascertain their presence or absence in selecting among health care providers. These leaps are a practical first step in using purchasing power to improve hospital safety and quality.

Leapfrog's member companies agree to adhere to the following four purchasing principles in buying health care for their enrollees:
1. Educating and informing enrollees about the safety, quality, and affordability of health care and the importance of comparing the care health care providers give. Initial emphasis on the Leapfrog safety and quality practices.
2. Recognizing and rewarding health care providers for major advances in the safety, quality, and affordability of their care.
3. Holding health plans accountable for implementing the Leapfrog purchasing principles.
4. Building the support of benefits consultants and brokers to use and advocate for the Leapfrog purchasing principles with all of their clients.

Source: Used with permission from The Leapfrog Group. 2005. "Factsheet." [Online information; retrieved 10/14/05.] www.leapfroggroup.org/about_us/leapfrog-factsheet.

throw it away in the nearest trash can. This manager's action exemplifies the principle of continuous improvement. While other hospital employees might walk past the trash, the environmental services manager realizes the importance of being committed to continuous improvement for her department and for the hospital; if at any time the manager sees something that needs fixing, improving, or correcting, she would take the initiative. If managers want to achieve continuous improvement in their organizations, they must demonstrate continuous improvement through their everyday actions.

Managerial Functions

The principle of continuous improvement may also be expressed through managers' execution of their managerial functions. For example, managers operating from this principle consider a performance measurement system an essential tool. This system includes indicators reported at various time intervals, depending on the nature of the work and the scope of management responsibility. For example, a shift supervisor for the patient transportation service in an 800-bed academic medical center watches the electronic dispatch system that displays a minute-by-minute update on transportation requests, indicators of patients en route to their destination, and the number of patients in the queue. By monitoring the system, the supervisor is immediately aware if a problem occurs and, as a result, is able to take action quickly to resolve the problem. If the number of requests unexpectedly increases, the supervisor can reassign staff breaks to maximize staff availability and minimize response times.

Each day, the supervisor posts the total number of transports performed the previous day along with the average response times. This way, the patient transporters are aware of the department's statistics and their own individual statistics, and this helps the transporters take pride in a job that is typically underappreciated by others in the organization. The daily performance data also enable the supervisor to quickly identify documented complaints and to address them within 24 hours, which in turn increases employee accountability and improves customer relations. On a monthly basis, the department manager and the shift supervisors review the volume of requests by hour of the day to determine if employees are scheduled appropriately to meet demand. The manager also reviews the statistics sorted by patient unit (e.g., nursing unit, radiology department) to identify any issues that need to be explored directly, manager to manager. The manager reviews the monthly statistics with his administrator, and the annual statistics are used in the budgeting process.

A performance measurement and management system such as this enables managers to continually monitor performance; to identify quality issues and performance gaps and to take action to resolve them; and to provide a foundation for ongoing communication, planning, and accountability.

Principle 3: Teamwork

In many organizations, when the terms "teamwork" and "quality" are used together, they usually refer to cross-functional or interdisciplinary project teams. When thinking about the principle of teamwork in relation to quality management, managers should also consider the philosophies and approaches used in carrying out functions inherent in the managerial role.

Organizational Philosophy

In the old days, when a physician entered the hospital unit, nurses were accustomed to offering their chairs to the physician because the nurses held lower positions in the organizational and professional hierarchies. Remnants of this tradition (e.g., deferring to someone higher in the hierarchy, ordering about someone lower in the hierarchy) may still be seen in healthcare organizations that operate from a bureaucratic philosophy.

An academic medical center, for example, may operate from a bureaucratic philosophy represented by multiple and parallel hierarchies. The CEO and the administrative team occupy the top positions in the management hierarchy, and frontline supervisors occupy the bottom. The department chairs are at the top of the medical staff hierarchy, and the interns or medical students are at the bottom. Physicians, followed by nurses, are at the top of the professional hierarchy, whereas other professionals (e.g., social workers, occupational therapists) all hold nondescript places lower in the hierarchy. Physicians and nurses hold the top spots in the jobs hierarchy, and the hourly manual laborers (e.g., environmental services and food service workers) are designated to the lower spots.

Although each group performs its respective duties in a competent manner, a lack of coordination among the groups and a lack of a common patient care approach can be observed. For example, physician teams typically make their morning patient rounds while nurses are occupied with the change-of-shift report. As a result, the nurses and physicians caring for the same patients rarely talk to each other during the course of day-to-day patient care.

The hospital can demonstrate many examples of CQI team projects; however, its teams tend to have an exclusive makeup (e.g., physician teams or nurse teams). Even though departments, such as the laboratory, have attempted on numerous occasions to create improvement teams with a mix of different providers, they have had little success in crossing the rigid boundaries of the professional and job hierarchies in the organization. Although the hospital is able to identify many teams, only a few examples of teamwork across and within these hierarchies can be seen.

The way philosophies and attitudes toward hierarchy and teamwork affect patient care and care teams is gaining more attention in the patient-safety discourse. "A distinguished neurosurgeon persists in operating on the wrong side of a woman's brain, in spite of vague protests by a resident who is aware of the error. In another hospital operating room, a surgeon and anesthesiologist resolve their differences by fisticuffs while an elderly patient lies anesthetized on the table" (Helmreich 1997, 67).

Situations such as these have prompted healthcare professionals to turn to other industries for strategies to promote more effective communication and teamwork. Survey instruments, training programs (e.g., Crew Resource Management), and operational interventions (e.g., daily briefings) provide managers of health services organizations with tools to better understand and minimize harm to patients as a result of healthcare's long history of professional hierarchy (Sexton, Thomas, and Helmreich 2000; Thomas, Sherwood, and Helmreich 2003; Miller 2005)

Managerial Functions

The manner by which management functions are implemented may promote or unintentionally discourage teamwork within the organization. The relationship between teamwork and three managerial functions—organizational design, resource allocation, and communication—is discussed in this section.

Organizational Design

Organizational design has been identified as a critical management function and encompasses "how the building blocks of the organization (authority, responsibility, accountability, information, and rewards) are arranged and rearranged to improve effectiveness and adaptive capacity" (Shortell and Kaluzny 2000, 275). The principle of teamwork implies that managers should proactively and purposefully arrange the organization's building blocks at all levels—individual positions, work groups, departmental, organizational—in a manner that supports teamwork.

Although the concept of high-performance work teams is not new in other industries (Hackman and Oldman 1980), the application of these lessons to the healthcare delivery setting is relatively recent. Nelson and colleagues have studied high-performing, frontline clinical teams in various healthcare settings and offer insights into success factors for designing a clinical microsystem to enhance quality outcomes and patient safety (Nelson et al. 2002; Mohr and Batalden 2002). A clinical microsystem is defined as a "group of clinicians and staff working together with a shared clinical purpose to provide care for a population of patients" (Mohr, Batalden, and Barach 2006). High-performing microsystems are characterized by "constancy of purpose, investment in improvement, alignment of role and training for efficiency and staff satisfaction, interdependence of care team to meet patient needs, integration of information and technology into work flows, ongoing measurement of outcomes, supportiveness of the larger organization, connection to the community to enhance care delivery and extend influence" (Mohr, Batalden, and Barach 2006). Upon closer examination, one sees that these characteristics result from intentional role and team design.

Some organizational designs, such as a matrix structure or a service-line structure, may promote teamwork. A matrix structure is characterized by a dual-authority system. In a service-line structure, a single person is responsible for all aspects of a group of services, usually based on patient type (e.g., pediatric, women's services, oncology, transplant services) (Shortell and Kaluzny 2000).

One large hospital used a hybrid of these two structures in its approach to organizational design. Each administrator was responsible for multiple departments that cared for patients with similar needs. For example, the trauma administrator was responsible for the emergency department, the trauma intensive care unit, and the air transport service. Although finance, human resources, and quality resources operated from their own centralized departments to maintain their unique competencies, each administrator in the hospital was assigned finance, human resources, and quality "consultants." Teamwork between the administrators and the dedicated staff consultants enhanced the staff's ability to provide consistent and responsive service to both the administrators and the managers for whom they were responsible.

Resource Allocation

Promoting effective interdependence between care team members implies the need for trust and understanding among team members. It is difficult to build working relationships in environments that experience high turnover and/or are staffed with continuous streams of temporary employees. While in the past, activities such as recruitment and retention might have fallen under the responsibilities of the human resources department, managers today must be keenly aware of the way human resources issues affect their ability not only to fulfill the quality-management principle of teamwork but also to promote quality patient outcomes and cost effectiveness.

A growing body of evidence links physician, nurse, and pharmacist staffing with patient outcomes in the hospital setting (Aiken et al. 2002; Bond, Rachl, and Frank 2001; Bond, Rachl, and Frank 2002; Dimick 2005; Hall, Doran, and Pink 2004; Needleman et al. 2002; Newhouse et al. 2005; Pronovost et al. 2002; Whitman et al. 2002). For example, levels and types of nurse staffing in hospitals have been linked with mortality rates (Aiken et al. 2002), medication errors, and wound infections (Hall, Doran, and Pink 2004); hospital lengths of stay, urinary tract infections, and pneumonia (Needleman et al. 2002); and "failure to rescue," which is defined as "death from pneumonia, shock or cardiac arrest, gastro-intestinal bleeding, sepsis, or deep vein thrombosis" (Aiken et al. 2002; Needleman et al. 2002). Central-line blood-associated infections, pressure ulcers, falls, medication errors, and use of restraints are considered "nurse-sensitive" outcomes (Whitman et al. 2002).

Human resources allocation decisions can be costly in terms of patient outcomes and also in terms of when the organization must fill and/or operate with staff vacancies. Filling a vacant position for a registered nurse can cost a healthcare organization between $42,000 and $67,000 (Aiken et al. 2002; Jones 2005), and organizational turnover costs have been estimated between 3.4 percent and 5.8 percent of the annual operating budget at one large, academic medical center (Waldman et al. 2004). When one considers that in 2004, U.S. hospital vacancy rates were 8.1 percent for registered nurses, 7.4 percent for pharmacists, 6.7 percent for licensed practical nurses, 6.7 percent for nursing assistants, 5.4 percent for imaging technicians, and 5 percent for lab technicians (American Hospital Association and the Lewin Group 2005), managers may appreciate the important role of effective resource allocation in quality management.

Communication   Improving communication between clinical care providers is a theme throughout JCAHO's NPSGs shown in Table 2.1. Designing and implementing decision making, documentation, and communication processes (which ensure individuals and teams have the information they need, when they need it, to make effective and timely clinical and organizational decisions) reflect a manager's understanding of the quality management principles.

For example, in one hospital, the manager of the materials management department negotiates with a supplier to obtain surgical gloves at a discounted rate, compared to the rate of the current supplier; the decision is made based on vendor and financial input. The first time the new gloves are used, however, the surgeon rips out the fingers of the gloves while inserting his hand. Had the manager embraced the concept of teamwork in her approach to decision making, she would have sought out information and input from the patient care team—the people who actually use the product and know the advantages and disadvantages of different brands of gloves.

Conclusion

This chapter begins an exploration of how the three principles of total quality—customer focus, continuous improvement, and teamwork—influence the way managers carry out their respective roles and functions. Although the examples provided in this chapter only begin to mention the implications for managers, the examples raise managers' awareness that their decisions and actions affect their ability to implement these principles throughout their entire organization. Readers are encouraged to continuously question how they can integrate the principles of total quality into decisions and activities inherent in their roles as managers. The exercise at the end of this chapter is designed to assist the readers to identify additional management behaviors and approaches that express the three principles of total quality. An overview of tools commonly used to implement the principle of continuous improvement is presented in Chapter 3.

Companion Readings

Aiken, L. H., S. P. Clark, D. M. Sloane, J. Sochalski, and J. H. Silber. 2002. "Hospital Nurse Staffing and Patient Mortality, Nurse Burnout, and Job Dissatisfaction." *JAMA* 288: 1987–93.

Dimick, J. B. 2005. "Organizational Characteristics and the Quality of Surgical Care." *Current Opinion in Critical Care* 11: 345–48.

Web Resources

Agency for Healthcare Research and Quality Patient Safety Network: A National Patient Safety Resource: www.psnet.ahrq.gov/index.aspx

The Joint Commission on Accreditation of Healthcare Organizations: www.jointcommission.org

The Joint Commission International Center for Patient Safety: www.jcipatientsafety.org

The Joint Commission National Patient Safety Goals: www.jointcommission.org/PatientSafety/NationalPatientSafetyGoals

The Leapfrog Group: www.leapfroggroup.org

National Committee for Quality Assurance: www.ncqa.org

National Patient Safety Foundation: www.npsf.org

The National Quality Forum: www.qualityforum.org

The University of Texas Human Factors Research Project: homepage.psy.utexas.edu/homepage/group/HelmreichLAB

References

Aiken, L. H., S. P. Clark, D. M. Sloane, J. Sochalski, and J. H. Silber. 2002. "Hospital Nurse Staffing and Patient Mortality, Nurse Burnout, and Job Dissatisfaction." *JAMA* 288: 1987–93.

American Hospital Association and the Lewin Group. 2005. *The Costs of Caring: Sources of Growth in Spending for Hospital Care.* Chicago: American Hospital Association.

Bond, C. A., C. L. Rachl, and T. Frank. 2001. "Medication Errors in United States Hospitals." *Pharmacotherapy* 21: 1023–36.

———. 2002. "Clinical Pharmacy Services, Hospital Pharmacy Staffing, and Medication Errors in United States Hospitals." *Pharmacotherapy* 22: 134–47.

Dean, J. W., and D. E. Bowen. 1994. "Management Theory and Total Quality: Improving Research and Practice Through Theory Development." *Academy of Management Review* 19: 392–418.

Devers, K. J., H. H. Pham, and G. Liu. 2004. "What Is Driving Hospitals' Patient Safety Efforts?" *Health Affairs* 23 (2): 103–15.

Dimick, J. B. 2005. "Organizational Characteristics and the Quality of Surgical Care." *Current Opinion in Critical Care* 11: 345–48.

Hackman, J. R., and G. R. Oldman. 1980. *Work Redesign.* Reading, MA: Addison-Wesley Publishing Company.

Hall, L. M., D. Doran, and G. H. Pink. 2004. "Nurse Staffing Models, Nursing Hours and Patient Safety Outcomes." *Journal of Nursing Administration* 34 (1): 41–45.

Helmreich, R. L. 1997. "Managing Human Error in Aviation." *Scientific American* 276 (5): 62–67.

James, B. C. 1989. *Quality Management for Healthcare Delivery.* Chicago: The Health Research and Educational Trust of the American Hospital Association.

Joint Commission on Accreditation of Healthcare Organizations. 2004. "National Patient Safety Goals, Hospitals." [Online information; retrieved 10/14/05.] www.jcipatientsafety.org/show.asp?durki=9738&site=164&return=9345.

———. 2005. "Facts About the 2005 National Patient Safety Goals." [Online information; retrieved 5/2/06.] www.jointcommission.org/PatientSafety/NationalPatientSafetyGoals/06_npsg_facts.htm.

———. 2006. "National Patient Safety Goals, Critical Access Hospital." [Online information; retrieved 5/2/06.] www.jcipatientsafety.org/show.asp?durki=10289.

Jones, C. B. 2005. "The Costs of Nursing Turnover, Part 2: Application of the Nursing Turnover Cost Calculation Methodology." *Journal of Nursing Administration* 35 (1): 41–49.

The Leapfrog Group. 2005. "Factsheet." [Online information; retrieved 10/14/05.] www.leapfroggroup.org/about_us/leapfrog-factsheet.

Miller, L. A. 2005. "Patient Safety and Teamwork in Perinatal Care: Resources for Clinicians." *Journal of Perinatal and Neonatal Nursing* 19 (1): 46–51.

Mohr, J. J., and P. B. Batalden. 2002. "Improving Safety on the Frontlines: The Role of Clinical Microsystems." *Quality and Safety in Health Care* 11: 45–50.

Mohr, J. J., P. Batalden, and P. Barach. 2006. "Inquiring into the Quality and Safety of Care in the Academic Clinical Microsystem." In *Continuous Quality Improvement in Health Care: Theory, Implementations, and Applications, 3rd edition*, edited by C. P. McLaughlin and A. D. Kaluzny, 281-96. Sudbury, MA: Jones and Bartlett Publishers.

National Institute for Standards and Technology. 2006. *Healthcare Criteria for Performance Excellence.* Washington, DC: National Institute for Standards and Technology.

Needleman, J., P. Buerhaus, S. Mattke, M. Stewart, and K. Zelevinsky. 2002. "Nurse-Staffing Levels and the Quality of Care in Hospitals." *New England Journal of Medicine* 346: 1715–22.

Nelson, E. C., P. B. Batalden, T. P. Huber, J. J. Mohr, M. M. Godfrey, L. A. Headrick, and J. H. Wasson. 2002. "Microsystems in Healthcare: Part 1. Learning from High-Performing Front-Line Clinical Units." *Joint Commission Journal on Quality Improvement* 28: 472–93.

Newhouse, R. P., M. Johantgen, P. J. Pronovost, and E. Johnson. 2005. "Perioperative Nurses and Patient Outcomes—Mortality, Complications, and Length of Stay." *Association of Operating Room Nurses Journal* 81: 508–09, 513–22, 525–28.

Pronovost, P. J., D. C. Angus, T. Dorman, K. A. Robinson, T. T. Dremsizov, and T. L. Young. 2002. "Physician Staffing Patterns and Clinical Outcomes in Critically Ill Patients: A Systematic Review." *JAMA* 288: 2151–62.

Sexton, J. B., E. J. Thomas, and R. L. Helmreich. 2000. "Error, Stress, and Teamwork in Medicine and Aviation: Cross Sectional Surveys." *British Medical Journal* 320: 745–49.

Shortell, S. M., and A. D. Kaluzny. 2000. *Healthcare Management: Organization Design and Behavior.* Albany, NY: Delmar Thomson Learning.

Thomas, E. J., G. D. Sherwood, and R. L. Helmreich. 2003. "Lessons from Aviation: Teamwork to Improve Patient Safety." *Nursing Economics* 21 (5): 241–43.

Waldman, J. D., F. Kelly, S. Aurora, and H. L. Smith. 2004. "The Shocking Cost of Turnover in Health Care." *Health Care Management Review* 29 (1): 2–7.

Whitman, G. R., Y. Kim, L. J. Davidson, G. A. Wolf, and S. Wang. 2002. "The Impact of Staffing on Patient Outcomes Across Specialty Units." *Journal of Nursing Administration* 32 (12): 633–39.

Exercise

This exercise may also be accessed on this book's companion website at ache.org/QualityManagement2.

Objective: To practice identifying management behaviors that express the three principles of total quality: customer focus, continuous improvement, and teamwork.

Instructions

1. Read the case study.
2. Describe at least one example of how management demonstrated the principle of customer focus in this case study.
3. Describe at least one example of how management demonstrated the principle of continuous improvement in this case study.
4. Describe at least one example of how management demonstrated the principle of teamwork in this case study.

Case Study

The following account of an improvement effort in an ambulatory surgery unit is told by the former *Wall Street Journal* columnist Thomas Petzinger, Jr.

While many companies are getting better at customer service, one industry has gotten a lot worse lately. That industry is medicine. The onslaught of managed care has commoditized what was once the most delicate relationship in all of commerce, that of doctor and patient. The practice of "capitation" creates the risk of a doctor visit becoming a cattle call. Accounting for the payment of services has overwhelmed the rendering of the services themselves. Yet a few islands of people have thrown off their Newtonian blinders and recognized that putting the customer first can redound to the benefit of the provider as well. With so many competing claims on every dollar, every process, and every hour of time and attention, the interests of the customer—the patient—serve as a common ground for making the entire system more efficient.

One hospital is such a place: a 520-bed teaching hospital and so-called trauma-one center with a stellar clinical reputation. Within the hospital, an outpatient surgery clinic was opened long ago, in which an ever-larger percentage of procedures were being conducted. And although the surgical staff was acclaimed, management recognized that the overall patient experience left something to be desired.

The main problem was delay. The surgery line was jam-packed as early as 5:30 every morning. Some patients spent the entire day lurching from check-in to pre-op to anesthesia to surgery to recovery to post-op, with too much of the time spent simply waiting. As much as some people may wish to convalesce at length as admitted hospital patients, no one wants to turn a four-hour outpatient experience into a nine-hour ordeal. If the hospital wanted to maintain (much less extend) its position in the marketplace, it had to figure out how to get patients through faster without degrading clinical results.

The job of facilitating the planning process went to an internal quality consultant who had worked for fifteen years as a registered nurse, mostly in neonatal intensive care, before earning her MBA and fulfilling this new organizational role. In her years in intensive care, she was often perplexed by the priorities that families exhibited in even the most dire medical situations. "I'm working like crazy to save a baby, but the parents get upset because the grandparents didn't get to see the baby!" she recalls. In time she could see that medicine was only part of health care. "Health care providers hold people's lives in their hands at a very vulnerable time," she says. "Health care is about a personal encounter." Most of the people on the business side of health care have little intellectual grasp and even less emotional grasp of this concept. Indeed, after moving to the business side herself, she became convinced that some of the most intractable problems of the industry could be solved only by people who, like her, combined far-flung disciplines. "Innovation will come from people who have crossed the boundaries from other disciplines," she says—from business to medicine, from medicine to law, and so on.

The facilitator insisted on involving the maximum number of nurses—people . . . who knew the whole patient as well as the individual surgeries they variously received. The new administrator over the area requested that the members of the improvement committee visit as many other hospitals as possible, within their large hospital system, to explore which outpatient surgical practices could be employed at their own site. And throughout the study process, the administrator continually harped on the "vision statement" of the initiative, which put as its first priority "to provide a patient/family focused quality culture."

This new administrator in the surgery service, a nurse herself, was a powerful force in leading the improvement effort. Under the previous leadership, the policy for change was simply "give the surgeons whatever they want," as she put it. The administrator acknowledged that the surgeon must call the shots on procedures—but not necessarily on process. In that respect she, too, insisted on using the patient as the point of departure. "If you're guided by only one phrase—what is best for the patient—you will always come up with the right answer," the administrator insists. (Hearing the administrator and facilitator say this over and over began to remind me of the best editors I have worked for. When in doubt, they would often say, do only what's right for the reader. Everything else will fall into place.)

Studying the surgery line from the patients' point of view was disturbingly illuminating. Surgeons showing up late for the first round of surgeries at 7:30 a.m. threw off the schedule for the entire day. The various hospital departments—admitting, financing, lab, surgery—all conducted their own separate interaction with the patient on each of their individual schedules. A poor physical layout, including a long corridor separating the operating rooms from pre-op, compounded the inefficiencies. Once a patient was called to surgery, he spent forty minutes waiting for an orderly to arrive with a wheelchair or gurney. And, because this was an outpatient surgery center located inside a hospital, the anesthesiologists were accustomed to administering heavy sedation, often slowing the patient's recovery from otherwise minor surgery and further clogging the entire line. The operation was a success, but the patient was pissed.

In talking to patients, the researchers discovered a subtext in the complaints about delays: resentment over the loss of personal control. Patients spent the day in God-awful gauze gowns, stripped of their underwear, their backsides exposed to the world. Partly this reflected a medical culture that considered the procedure, not the patient, as the customer. As the administrator put it to me, "If you're naked on a stretcher on your back, you're pretty subservient." Family members, meanwhile, had to roam the hospital in search of change so they could coax a cup of coffee from a vending machine. She marveled at the arrogance of it. "You're spending $3,000 on a loved one, but you'd better bring correct change."

Fortunately, this administrator had the political standing to push through big changes, and although the staff surgeons effectively had veto power, most were too busy to get very deeply involved in the improvement process. Because few patients enjoy getting stuck with needles, the nurses created a process for capturing the blood from the insertion of each patient's intravenous needle and sending it to the lab for whatever tests were necessary. This cut down not only on discomfort, but on time, money and scheduling complexity. The unremitting bureaucratic questions and paperwork were all replaced with a single registration packet that patients picked up in their doctors' offices and completed days before ever setting foot in the hospital; last-minute administrative details were attended to in a single phone call the day before surgery. The nurses set up a check-in system for the coats and valuables of patients and family members, which eliminated the need for every family to encamp with their belongings in a pre-op room for the entire day. A family-friendly waiting area was created, stocked with free snacks and drinks. There would be no more desperate searches for correct change.

That was only the beginning. Patients had always resented having to purchase their post-op medications from the hospital pharmacy; simply freeing them to use their neighborhood drugstore got them out of the surgery line sooner, further relieving the congestion. Also in the interest of saving time, the nurses made a heretical proposal to allow healthy outpatients to walk into surgery under their own power, accompanied by their family members, rather than waiting forty minutes for a wheelchair or gurney. That idea got the attention of the surgeons, who after years of paying ghastly malpractice premiums vowed that the administrator, not they, would suffer the personal liability on that one. The risk-management department went "eek" at the idea. Yet as the improvement committee pointed out, the hospital permitted outpatients to traverse any other distance in the building by foot. Why should the march into surgery be any different?

In a similar vein, the nurses suggested allowing patients to wear underwear beneath their hospital gowns. The administrators could scarcely believe their ears: "Show me one place in the literature where patients wear underwear to surgery!" one top administrator demanded. (The nurses noted that restricting change to what had been attempted elsewhere would automatically eliminate the possibility of any breakthrough in performance.) And why stop at underwear, the nurses asked. The hospital was conducting more and more outpatient cataract operations; why not let these patients wear their clothes into surgery? "Contamination!" the purists cried. But clothing is no dirtier than the skin beneath it, the nurses answered. This change eliminated a major post-op bottleneck caused by elderly patients who could not dress themselves or tie their shoes with their heads clouded by anesthesia and their depth perception altered by the removal of their cataracts.

As the changes took effect, the nurses observed another unintended effect. Patients were actually reducing their recovery times! People were no longer looking at ceiling tiles on their way into surgery like characters in an episode of *Dr. Kildare*. They went into surgery feeling better and came out of it feeling better. In case after case they were ready to leave the joint faster, which in turn freed up even more space for other patients. Because they had studied practices at a number of stand-alone clinics, the nurses even suggested to the physicians that the outpatients would be better off with less anesthesia, hastening their recoveries, speeding their exit, and freeing up still more capacity.

Within a year, the volume at the outpatient surgery unit had surged 50 percent with no increase in square footage and no increase in staff. Customer-service surveys were positive and costs were under control. And it dawned on the facilitator that the nurses' intuitive conviction that the patient should come first benefited the surgery line itself at every single step. Everyone and everything connected to the process—surgeon, staff, insurers, time, cost, and quality—seemed to come out ahead when the patients' interests came first.

What was really happening, of course, was that the change teams simply put common sense first. In a complex process of many players, the interest of the patient was the one unifying characteristic—the best baseline for calibration—because the patient was the only person touched by every step.

Reprinted with slight changes, with the permission of Simon & Schuster Adult Publishing Group from *The New Pioneers: The Men and Women Who Are Transforming the Workplace and Marketplace* by Thomas Petzinger, Jr. Copyright © 1999 by Thomas Petzinger, Jr.

THE MANAGER'S TOOLBOX

OBJECTIVES

* To introduce commonly used continuous improvement and patient-safety tools
* To practice using continuous improvement and patient safety tools

An employee is faced with choosing a new primary care physician when her employer changes health plans. This employee makes a list of the characteristics she wants in a physician (e.g., board certified) and in the physician's office (e.g., close to work). She asks fellow employees and friends if they know any of the physicians listed in the health plan handbook and what they think of their care experiences. She then selects a physician and makes an appointment for an annual physical. After her first experience with the new physician, she decides that both the physician and the office staff meet her criteria and that she will continue to use the physician as her primary care physician.

Although this employee may not have realized it, the continuous-improvement approach used in her organization had "rubbed off" on her so that she automatically used the same systematic process for deciding what to do when faced with a personal problem or decision. She planned how to select a physician; collected data about her options; compared the various options against her criteria; tested her first choice; and, based on her impressions and experiences, decided to keep her first choice as her primary care physician. She had used a variation of what is referred to in the quality improvement literature as the Shewhart cycle (Figure 3.1).

Originating from industrial applications of quality improvement, the Shewhart cycle (also referred to as the PDCA cycle) consists of four steps: planning, doing, checking/studying, and acting. The steps are linked to represent the cyclical nature of the approach. In the planning step, the process of concern is investigated and studied to better understand the problem(s) and to identify how to improve the process. In the doing step, the new process or intervention is implemented on a small scale to test its effectiveness. The checking/studying step involves monitoring the results of the intervention to determine how well the new process is working. Finally, in the acting step, the results and effects are reviewed to determine

FIGURE 3.1

Shewhart
Cycle

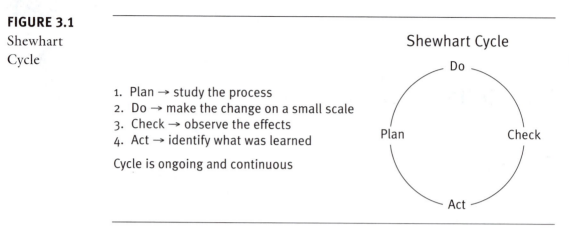

Shewhart Cycle

1. Plan → study the process
2. Do → make the change on a small scale
3. Check → observe the effects
4. Act → identify what was learned

Cycle is ongoing and continuous

Source: Reprinted with permission from Deming, W. E. 2000. *Out of the Crisis,* p. 88. Cambridge, MA: The MIT Press. © MIT Press.

what was learned from the small-scale trial. On the basis of what was learned from the test, the new process is studied and refinements are made, and this second planning step begins the cycle again.

Why is a systematic approach to improvement as represented by the Shewhart cycle important? The Shewhart cycle offers a framework to incorporate the scientific method into improvement approaches. Employees at all levels of an organization—from entry level to the executive suite—may use this simple four-step process to promote problem solving in the work setting.

Clinical providers are trained in the scientific method in their approaches to clinical problem solving. First, patients present with some kind of problem. Clinicians then gather subjective data (what the patients tell them) and objective data (e.g., vital signs, physical exam, diagnostic tests); devise a patient plan based on the data (e.g., select a medication); implement the plan (e.g., order drugs and educate the patient); evaluate the plan (e.g., collect additional subjective and objective data and compare to previous data); and revise the plan as needed (e.g., increase or decrease dosage or change to new drug). When clinical professionals use the scientific method in decision making, it is often referred to as "professional judgment" (Facione et al. 2005).

Likewise, managerial professional judgment may be described by the concept of *critical thinking.* Why is critical thinking the foundation for the manager's toolbox? "Everyone thinks; it is our nature to do so. But much of our thinking, left to itself, is biased, distorted, partial, uninformed or down-right prejudiced. Yet the quality of our life and that of what we produce, make, or build depends precisely on the quality of our thought. Shoddy thinking is costly, both in money and in quality of life. Excellence in thought, however, must be systematically cultivated" (Critical Thinking Community 2005).

The broader the scope of responsibility managers have in the health services organization, the greater the imperative to develop, cultivate, and refine their critical thinking skills. Critical thinking is essential if managers are to be effective stewards of limited human and financial resources as well as the patients' lives and health that are entrusted to their organizations or their community.

A manager who exhibits effective critical thinking (Critical Thinking Community 2005) does the following:

- "raises vital questions and problems, formulating them clearly and precisely;
- gathers and assesses relevant information, using abstract ideas to interpret it effectively, comes to well-reasoned conclusions and solutions, testing them against relevant criteria and standards;
- thinks open-mindedly within alternative systems of thought, recognizing and assessing, as need be, their assumptions, implications, and practical consequences; and
- communicates effectively with others in figuring out solutions to complex problems."

Managers may begin to cultivate their critical thinking skills by consistently asking the following three questions when faced with a problem or performance gap (Langley et al. 1996, 10):

1. What are we trying to accomplish?
2. How will we know that a change is an improvement?
3. What change can we make that will result in an improvement?

Just as clinical providers use tools to aid in their process of clinical judgment, managers must take advantage of the numerous tools available to assist them in their critical-thinking processes. This chapter will discuss two categories of tools: those that are used in an improvement effort and those that help promote patient safety.

Improvement Tools

Often an organization may select and endorse a particular improvement technique found in the quality improvement literature (Institute for Healthcare Improvement 2003; Juran 1989; Langley et al. 1996; Scholtes, Joiner, and Streibel 2003; Walton 1986). Managers will find the following common steps in these techniques: systematically identifying causes of problems, designing and implementing improvements, and monitoring and continually improving the effects of the intervention. The tools presented in this chapter will assist managers as they approach continuous improvement within the context of their own organization's preferred technique.

Tools for CQI focus a team's problem-solving efforts and provide a document trail that managers may use to organize and record the improvement process and results of the project intervention(s). Documentation is essential to ensure continuity between project meetings and to provide a mechanism for sharing knowledge, promoting ongoing learning, encouraging follow-up on outcomes, and building team confidence through a concrete display of the team's accomplishments.

Improvement tools fall into four general categories:

1. Identifying customer and stakeholder expectations
2. Documenting a process
3. Diagnosing the problem
4. Monitoring progress

For readers who desire a more comprehensive description of the tools presented below, please refer to the references and web resources at the end of this chapter.

Identifying Customer Expectations

As described in Chapter 2, customer focus is one of the three principles of quality management. Identifying and understanding customer expectations and requirements are essential components of this principle. Asking and observing are the most informal ways to identify patient needs and expectations. Scanning the published literature for information on customer expectations can help a manager avoid reinventing the wheel. For example, the Picker Institute was established in 1987 to promote patient-focused care and to provide information to healthcare organizations about patient-focused approaches. On the basis of information obtained from focus groups, literature, and health professionals, the Picker Institute has identified and defined specific patient requirements, also called dimensions of care (Gerteis et al. 1993; NRC+Picker 2005):

- Respect for patients' values, preferences, and expressed needs
- Coordination and integration of care
- Information and education
- Physical comfort
- Emotional support and alleviation of fear and anxiety
- Involvement of family and friends
- Transition and continuity
- Access to care

These dimensions of care described by the NRC+Picker provide an excellent starting point for any healthcare manager to begin a customer-focused improvement effort. Depending on the organization's needs and resources, a deeper understanding of patient requirements may be obtained through focus groups and other qualitative research methods.

Once patient expectations are known, they must be translated into product or service features to ensure that they are being met on a consistent basis for all customers who interact with that product or service. As consumers, many readers are already acquainted with this concept. Internet banking is one example of how financial organizations have created new service features to meet customer expectations for convenient, low-hassle banking services. Experienced healthcare organizations are continually improving their abilities to translate patient expectations into service and product features.

For example, most healthcare providers and employees would describe themselves as "caring"; however, what does caring mean, and how is it expressed by all employees who interact with patients? In one multiphysician practice, caring is defined by the following behaviors: calling patients by name, looking at patients when talking to them, escorting patients to the examination rooms, explaining to patients what they can expect during the visit, and explaining to patients the reasons for any delays experienced during the visit. Office staff (i.e., receptionists, nurses, business office employees, and physicians) are trained and expected to demonstrate these behaviors. In this way, while allowing for individual staff styles and personalities, the practice ensures that all patients receive a consistent level of caring each time they visit the office.

Providers of women's specialty care have been particularly effective in translating customer expectations into service features because obstetrics patients have been vocal over the years about their needs and expectations of care providers and facilities. Managers responsible for other clinical areas may gain valuable insights from labor and delivery room design, visiting policies, and prenatal/postpartum education efforts. Labor and delivery processes may help managers better understand the concept of translating patient requirements into actual service features and product design (see Table 3.1).

Health services organizations use a variety of sources, such as market research, professional associations, journals, published studies, news abstract services, and business contracts, to keep up-to-date on stakeholder requirements. Like patient expectations, once stakeholder requirements are identified, organizational processes, functions, and service features must then be designed and/or improved to ensure that the requirements are being met. Chapter 2 provided examples of requirements from two key stakeholders: JCAHO and The Leapfrog Group.

Documenting a Process

Some of the most valuable improvement tools are those that help managers and teams better understand work processes. It is not uncommon to carry out a process because "that is how we have always done it" or because a certain way of doing things has simply evolved over time. Before a process can be improved, understanding what the current process entails is essential. Using any of the tools described in this section not only provides the opportunity to document the process but also to discuss, question, and clarify perceptions or misconceptions about the process.

TABLE 3.1
Translating
Customer
Requirements
Into Service
Features
(Example:
Women's
Service)

Customer Requirement (Picker Dimension of Care)	Service/Product Feature
Involvement of family and friends	Postpartum or labor/delivery/recovery room size is large enough to accommodate more than one visitor
	Furniture in patient rooms includes a pullout sofa or cot for father/significant other
	Policies designed for flexible and "safe" visiting hours for grandparents, siblings, and friends (e.g., after screening for infectious illness)
Transition and continuity	Hospital preregistration in advance of admission
	Prenatal and postpartum educational offerings
	Follow-up nurse phone calls

A process is "a set of causes and conditions that repeatedly come together in a series of steps to transform inputs into outcomes" (Langley et al. 1996, 20). Benefits of documenting a process include the following:

- Providing a visual picture of the process
- Distinguishing the distinct steps of the process
- Identifying unnecessary steps in the process
- Understanding vulnerabilities—where breakdowns, mistakes, or delays are likely to occur—in a process
- Detecting rework loops that contribute to inefficiency and quality waste

Three tools for documenting processes are described in this section: a process flowchart, a workflow diagram, and lead-time analysis.

Process Flowchart

A process flowchart is a picture of the sequence of steps in a process. Different steps are represented by different-shaped symbols. An oval indicates the start and end of the process, a rectangle indicates a process action step, and a diamond indicates a decision that must be made in the process. Depending on the decision, the process follows different paths.

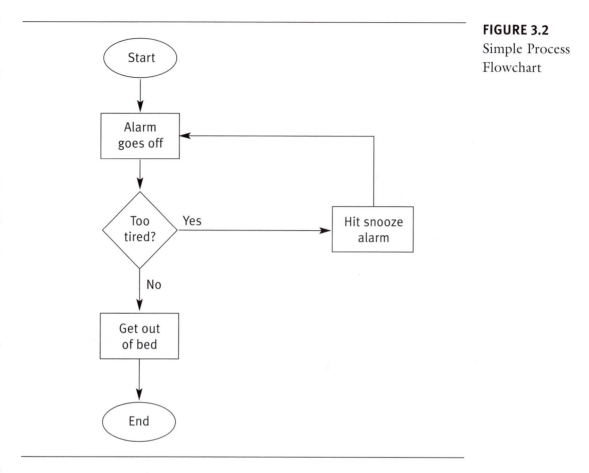

FIGURE 3.2

Simple Process
Flowchart

Figure 3.2 illustrates an example of a simple flowchart that documents the process of getting out of bed in the morning. The oval labeled "Start" indicates the beginning of the process. The first step in the process is represented by the rectangle labeled "Alarm goes off." The second step is a decision step represented by the diamond labeled "Too tired?" The steps are connected by arrows that indicate the relationships between the steps. If the answer to the question "Too tired?" is "No," then the next step is "Get out of bed," and the process ends. If the answer to the question "Too tired?" is "Yes," the process follows an alternate path to the step labeled "Hit snooze alarm," which in turn leads back to the first step in the process ("Alarm goes off"). This alternate path is referred to as a rework loop and may be a clue to inefficiencies or unnecessary duplication in the process. Clinicians may already be familiar with this tool, as many clinical algorithms and guidelines are communicated using process flowcharts.

An example of a clinical guideline flowchart is shown in Figure 3.3. This particular guideline is one of many developed by the Institute for Clinical Systems Improvement, a nonprofit organization that provides quality improvement services to medical groups in the state of Minnesota (Institute for

FIGURE 3.3

Institute for Clinical Systems Improvement Healthcare Guideline: Diagnosis and Treatment of ST Elevated Acute Myocardial Infarction

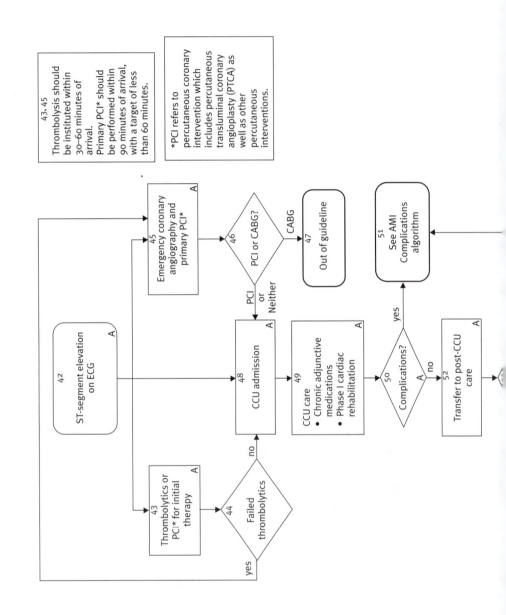

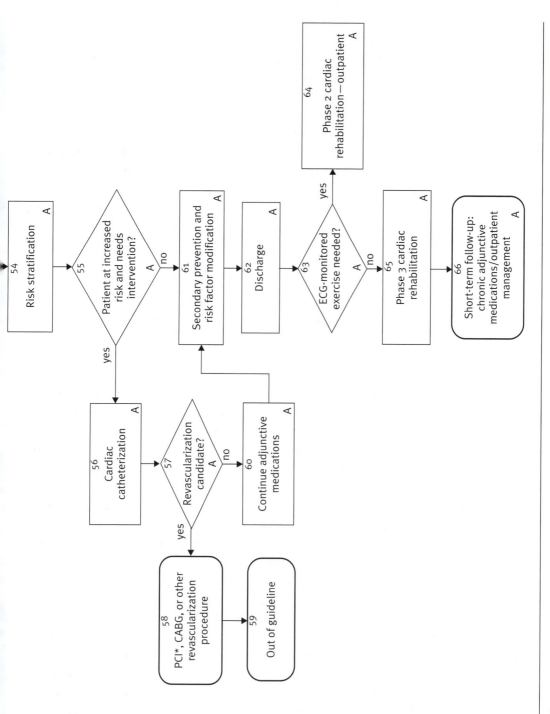

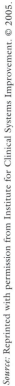

Clinical Systems Improvement 2003, 2005). The flowchart format displays the sequence of interventions, steps, and decisions that the clinical provider makes in evaluating and treating an acute myocardial infarction.

A deployment flowchart is useful when the steps in a single process are carried out by different people, departments, or organizations. Efforts to improve coordination of process steps may be enhanced by identifying, documenting, and understanding the essential handoffs that occur in a process. Figure 3.4 illustrates a deployment flowchart for a surgical procedure; in this example, the anesthesiologists wanted to reduce delays between surgical procedures. In a deployment flowchart, the steps in the process are documented with the same symbols used in a process flowchart. The columns in which the symbol is located represent the individual or group responsible for carrying out that step in the process. By using a deployment flowchart, steps occurring in parallel can be shown and so can the amount of time the patient spent with each member of the staff in the process, which is represented by the time labels (e.g., Time 1, Time 2) at the bottom of each column. In this way, delays can be readily tracked to their source and, in turn, targeted for improvement.

Workflow Diagram

A workflow diagram is a tool used to document how people or things actually move through the physical workspace. This tool is especially useful when it becomes difficult to "see the forest for the trees."

A workflow diagram was instrumental in improving patient flow in a redesign effort for an ambulatory surgery unit. The unit was an outpatient facility located within a tertiary care hospital. The unit location and design had been chosen to be close to a public entrance with automobile access; however, because other patients and staff also used this entrance, many got lost in the ambulatory surgery unit or used the unit as a thoroughfare to other destinations in the hospital. A common comment heard from nurses in the ambulatory surgery unit was, "Why does it feel as busy as an emergency department here?"

The nurse manager acquired an official floor plan from the maintenance and engineering department and began mapping the patient flow with simple lines. She found herself drawing long lines from the satellite laboratory that serviced the ambulatory surgery unit and was located at one end of the unit to the outside entrance that was located at the other end of the unit. Upon further investigation, she realized that the nonsurgical patient traffic had steadily increased over the years as physicians in the office complex across the street found it convenient to send their own patients to this satellite laboratory for testing. The nurse manager realized that this outpatient laboratory traffic was contributing to the hustle and bustle of activity normally felt only in higher-intensity areas such as the emergency department. Once the workflow diagram was completed, the solution became obvious: move the satellite laboratory from the end of the

FIGURE 3.4

Deployment Flowchart Example

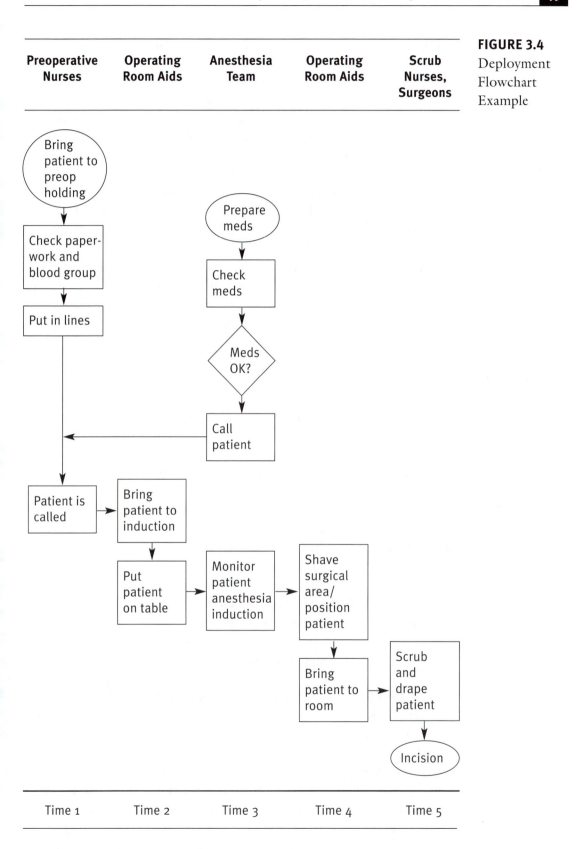

Preoperative Nurses	Operating Room Aids	Anesthesia Team	Operating Room Aids	Scrub Nurses, Surgeons

Bring patient to preop holding

Check paperwork and blood group

Put in lines

Prepare meds

Check meds

Meds OK?

Call patient

Patient is called

Bring patient to induction

Put patient on table

Monitor patient anesthesia induction

Shave surgical area/ position patient

Bring patient to room

Scrub and drape patient

Incision

Time 1	Time 2	Time 3	Time 4	Time 5

unit that was farthest from the outside entrance to the end of unit that was closest to the outside entrance.

A workflow diagram also proved useful in the redesign of a laboratory's services. The large laboratory consisted of many smaller specialty laboratories, such as chemistry, cytology, hematology, and bacteriology. Sometimes specimens went to a single area only; however, a specimen was often sent to multiple specialties that each took their portion of the sample and then passed it along to the next area. Early in the redesign process, the team used a workflow diagram to map the flow of specimens within the laboratory facility. The overlapping and backtracking lines drawn on the floor plan became affectionately known to the team as the "plate of spaghetti" (see Figure 3.5). Although the team had sensed that the location of the specialty laboratories in relation to each other was not quite right, the workflow diagram concretely illustrated the inefficiencies and unnecessarily complicated and confusing flow. In turn, ideas about how and where to relocate equipment and people to streamline flow and maximize efficiency became evident to the team members (Kelly 1998).

Lead-Time Analysis

Lead-time analysis, a tool used in General Motors' (GM) PICOS quality efforts, was taught to healthcare workers during collaborative efforts in which PICOS staff assisted hospitals in their improvement efforts (Pougnet 1996). The lead-time analysis tool (see Figure 3.6), like a workflow diagram, is useful in understanding the physical path taken during a process.

The user of this tool physically walks through the process that a document, a specimen, a piece of equipment, or a patient would follow. If a manager is using lead-time analysis to study the patient admission process, he or she would start at the same place as the patient by driving to the hospital parking garage. In the first column of the lead-time analysis (Step #), the steps of the process are numbered in sequence. In the second column (Process Step Description), the actual action that takes place at this point is described. The first step of the admission process, for example, may be described as "Drive around parking lot until an empty space is found."

The rest of the columns are then completed for the step: the time it takes to complete the step, the distance covered for that step or the distance between steps, the number of times that step occurs (during the process or throughout the day), and if the step adds value to the process. (GM defines value-added as "something that the customer is willing to pay for" [Pougnet 1996].)

Because in healthcare certain steps of a process may be dictated by a regulatory requirement, this adapted version of GM's lead-time analysis includes a column for regulatory requirements. Although a customer may not be willing to pay for this step of the process, it is essential that it remains. Another addition to the GM version of the tool is to evaluate the process step in relation to the organizational mission, vision, and values. Clearly,

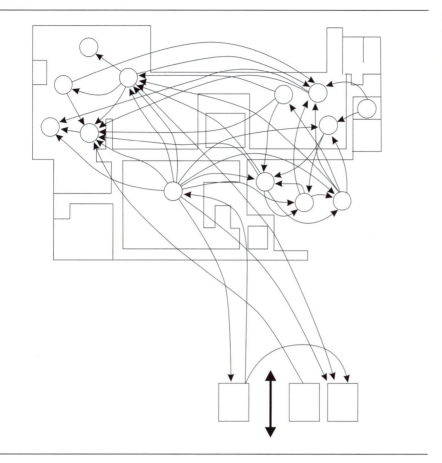

FIGURE 3.5
Workflow
Diagram
Example

the process step described in this patient admission example, where it took 15 minutes and three trips around the parking garage to find a parking place, is not aligned with an organization that tries to be patient focused.

As with the workflow diagram, the actual process of completing the tool, not just reviewing the information written on the form, often leads to identifying obvious areas for improvement. In the laboratory redesign effort described previously, the team also used the lead-time analysis tool. One team member completed it to better understand the journey taken by test results once she had finished analyzing a specimen. She knew she completed the analysis in a timely fashion and was baffled by the numerous complaints her specialty laboratory received about delayed results. The lead-time analysis revealed a cumbersome process that caused a printed laboratory result to make a three- to five-day journey through the interoffice mail system to the physicians' offices across the street. As she continued to explore the process, this technician found that this was the case for many of the smaller offices served by the laboratory. Although the larger clinics typically receive results more quickly, because they had a printer interface with the laboratory's information system, the smaller offices depended on

FIGURE 3.6
Lead-Time Analysis Grid

Process/Product Description _____ Page _____ of _____

Step #	Process Step Description	Time	Distance	Quantity	Value-added	Non-Value-added	Regulatory Requirement	Aligned with MVV
1	Drive around parking lot until an empty space is found	15 min.	0.5 mi.	3		✓	No	No

Date completed: _____ Prepared by: _____

Source: Reprinted with permission from General Motors Corporation, Warren, Michigan.

interoffice or postal service mail. When results were not received in a timely manner, an office staff member would usually call the laboratory and someone would have to look up and print the results and then fax the results to the caller. Documenting the process using the lead-time analysis revealed the duplication of work, the quality waste, and the source of delays before physicians and patients received their test results. Understanding the process helped the team identify and implement solutions to reduce delays in clinicians' receiving the test results (Kelly 1998).

Diagnosing the Problem

The following tools can help with the documentation, organization, and prioritization of possible causes of a problem: fishbone diagram, check sheet, and Pareto diagram.

Fishbone Diagram

A cause-and-effect diagram is a tool for identifying and organizing the possible causes of a problem in a structured format (Scholtes, Joiner, and Streibel 2003). Because this diagram resembles a fish (the problem represents the head and the causes represent the bones), it is also referred to as a fishbone diagram. The problem is written on the far right of the diagram. Categories of causes are represented by the diagonal lines (bones) connected to the horizontal line (spine), which leads to the problem (head). Figures 3.7 and 3.8 illustrate two common ways to draw and label a fishbone diagram.

Managers may also find it useful to label problems related to service processes according to the Four Ps: people, procedures, policies, and plant. Categories labeled with the Four Ms—manpower, materials, methods, and machinery—may be better suited for problems associated with production processes or technology. Once possible causes have been identified and documented, actual causes may be verified through further investigation and data collection.

Figure 3.9 is an example of a fishbone diagram used by a multidisciplinary improvement team charged with addressing the problem of inconsistent patient identification before rendering clinical services. In this example, the Four Ps were used as the general categories to organize the causes. Detailed causes are identified and represented by the small bones of the fish. Identification band and care issues may be found as a cause under the category labeled "People." When this cause is broken down further, three additional causes are documented: edema (swelling that may be related to the patient's clinical status), hidden (covered with sterile drapes in the operating room), and IV line (wristband interfering with site of IV line insertion or stabilization).

Check Sheet

Although many organizations have electronic systems from which to obtain data reports, smaller organizations or physician practices may be limited in their ability to collect data in electronic formats. Managers must remember that valuable information may be obtained using tools such as talking to

FIGURE 3.7

Fishbone
Diagram: The
Four Ps

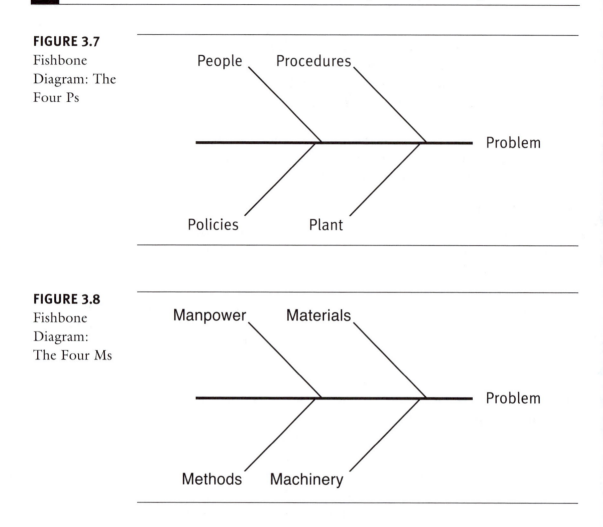

FIGURE 3.8

Fishbone
Diagram:
The Four Ms

employees and using pencil-and-paper data collection to better understand a problem. A check sheet is one of these "low tech" tools. A check sheet is "a simple data collection form on which you make hash marks to indicate how often something occurs" (Scholtes, Joiner, and Streibel 2003, 4-13).

Figure 3.10 shows an example of a check sheet used by an obstetrics and gynecology clinic to track different types of phone calls to the clinic. In this case, the clinic manager had been receiving numerous complaints from patients that they were unable to get through when phoning the clinic. Although the phone company could provide aggregate data helpful to evaluate productivity (e.g., number of total calls, average time on hold, number of interrupted calls [caller hanging up while on hold]), this type of information would not help the manager identify the cause or solve the patients' complaint. The manager's first step was to ask employees to identify the types of calls they received in a typical day. The manager then needed to collect data on the frequency of each of these types of calls. When employees are asked to collect data for a short period of time with the

FIGURE 3.9
Fishbone Diagram Example

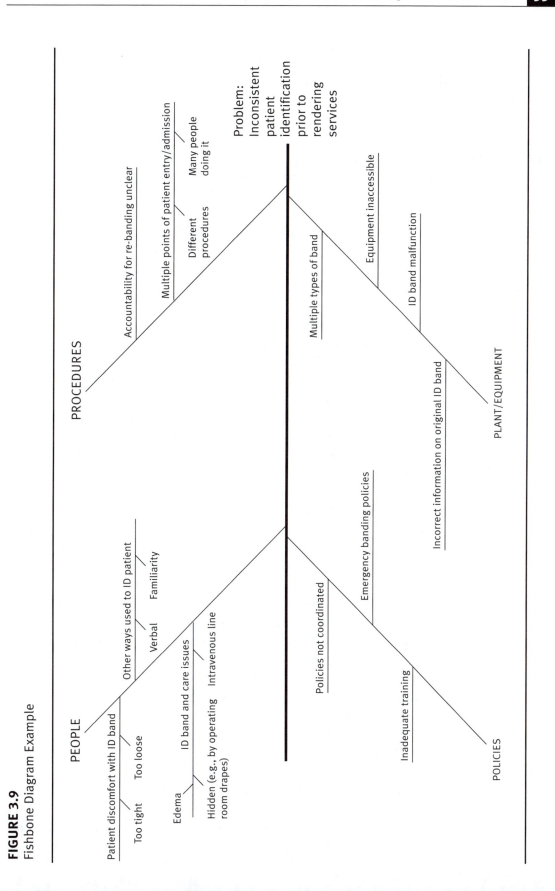

intent of addressing a work problem they are concerned with, they will typically consent to the request. The clinic's phone room staff were asked to complete the data-collection check sheet each day for a week.

A user-friendly check sheet should be easy to understand, accessible to the user, and simple enough to be completed quickly.

Pareto Chart   Once data about a problem have been collected, the manager may use a Pareto chart to help prioritize improvement interventions and focus activities on the highest leverage areas. A Pareto chart is a simple graph that displays data in descending order using a bar graph and displays cumulative totals using a line graph when reading from left to right. Figure 3.11 illustrates a Pareto chart for the data collected on the check sheet by the clinic's phone room staff. Graphing the data this way helped the clinic manager select specific interventions that would best address the problem.

First, the phone team members identified that, although the most frequent number of calls were about making appointments, not all of these calls actually resulted in an actual appointment being scheduled. Because the physicians provided their schedules 30 days in advance, any caller requesting or requiring an appointment beyond this time frame was asked to call back. A patient calling three times to obtain a single appointment was not uncommon. In addition, the time spent telling patients to call back could have been used for other purposes, thereby increasing the productivity of the phone room staff. Next, the manager was able to identify an unintended consequence of a previous intervention. In an effort to create a more patient-friendly clinic, intercom paging of the nurses and physicians had been eliminated. When the Pareto chart showed that calls for nurses and physicians accounted for about 25 percent of total calls, it helped explain why many patients could not get through in a timely way: callers were placed on hold for excessive amounts of time, while the phone room staff searched for nurses and doctors in this large clinic to notify them of their phone calls.

Readers may wonder why the manager needed a Pareto chart to discover this problem. An important lesson for managers who are beginning improvement efforts is to ensure that improving one problem in one area does not create a problem in a different area. In this case, a new medical director was very distressed by the noise and disruption of the pages. In an effort to satisfy the medical director, the manager did not think to implement an alternative method of communication between the phone staff and the clinical providers.

The second most frequent type of call fell under the category of "Other." For every two calls for an appointment, the phone room was receiving one "other" call, the purpose of which was not readily explained. This realization prompted the manager to further investigate the "other" category to gain insights into the type of calls interfering with appointment-generating calls or calls related to clinical questions. Rather than

FIGURE 3.10

Check Sheet Example

OB/GYN Phone Room
Data Collection Sheet: Volume of Calls by Type

Name _____   Day of the week:　M　T　W　Th　Fr

Type of Call	8:00–9:00 a.m.	9:01–10:00 a.m.	10:01–11:00 a.m.	11:01 a.m.–12:00 p.m.	12:01–1:00 p.m.	1:01–2:00 p.m.	2:01–3:00 p.m.	3:01–4:00 p.m.	4:01–5:00 p.m.
Make an appointment									
Call for nurse: patient									
Call for nurse: nonpatient									
Call for MD: patient									
Call for MD: nonpatient									
Personal call									
Wrong number									
Asking for a phone number									
Other									

Instructions: Please place a tic mark for each phone call you receive in the appropriate time and type box. Use the back of this sheet for comments and/or to describe reasons for "other" calls.

FIGURE 3.11
Pareto Chart
Example

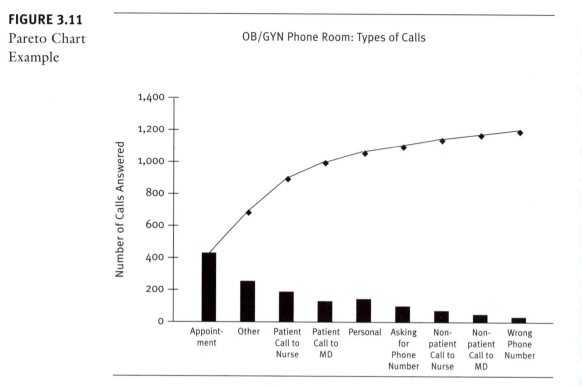

OB/GYN Phone Room: Types of Calls

lobby for more phone room staff, which was the solution proposed initially, the clinic manager set about negotiating with the physicians to receive their schedules further in advance, instituting an internal pager system to replace the overhead intercom, and identifying the reasons for the "other" phone calls.

Monitoring Progress

A run chart is a graphic representation of data over time; run charts help monitor progress after an improvement intervention and for ongoing operations. On a run chart, the x-axis represents the time interval (e.g., day, month, quarter, year) and the y-axis represents the variable of interest. Displaying data on a run chart also enables a manager to more readily detect patterns or unusual occurrences in the data.

Figure 3.12 illustrates a run chart showing monthly patient visits to a mammography center. For several months the center's staff had been complaining about being very busy. The manager needed to determine if the increase in visits was here to stay or if it was a passing phenomenon. She converted the volume statistics from a series of monthly management reports to a run chart and was then able to determine the answer to her question. A "once every hundred years" snowstorm had hit the city the previous January and literally shut down business for four days. The center's current busyness was a reflection of the need to

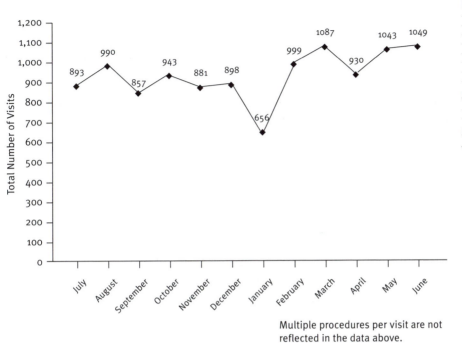

FIGURE 3.12

Run Chart
Example for
Breast
Imaging
Services:
Diagnostic and
Screening
Visits

Multiple procedures per visit are not
reflected in the data above.

reschedule appointments that were cancelled as a result of the snow-storm. The overall volumes for the year were still on track; it was the monthly distribution of visits that had been affected by this unusual and explainable event.

Figure 3.13 illustrates another example of a run chart. In this case, the internal medicine clinic of a large multispecialty physician practice implemented changes in its workflow to reduce patient waiting times and improve patient satisfaction. The run chart shows that patient satisfaction actually decreased the first month after the changes were implemented in September. This is not uncommon because new processes often take time to stabilize as a result of staff learning curves and adjustments. Managers must not overreact to one month's worth of data but should continue to track results over time to see the pattern of performance once the process has stabilized. This run chart demonstrates that although patient satisfaction dropped initially, in subsequent months it stabilized at a higher average level and that more consistent performance became apparent from month to month.

Patient Safety Tools

As patient safety gains prominence in the discourse on healthcare quality, new tools have emerged to supplement the traditional improvement tools.

FIGURE 3.13

Run Chart
Example for
Overall Patient
Satisfaction:
Internal
Medicine
Clinic

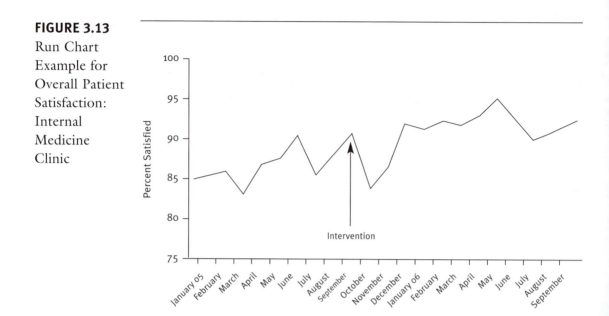

Understanding and improving the safety of processes may be thought of
from two perspectives. Problems may be anticipated and processes improved
to prevent problems from occurring, or actual problems may be investigated to better understand the problem and actions taken to prevent their
recurrence. The failure mode and effects analysis (FMEA) is a proactive,
preventive tool, whereas an in-depth root cause analysis is a retrospective,
investigative tool.

Failure Mode and Effects Analysis

Anyone who has lost documents and wasted hours of work in the early
days of personal computers can appreciate the periodic autosave, a pop-
up warning of a low battery, and the rescued document features that are
commonplace for users of contemporary personal computers or laptop
computers. These features illustrate computer designers' understanding
of the consequences of hardware and software failures on their users and
subsequently incorporating product designs that prevent the failure from
occurring (e.g., save the document before the battery runs out) or the
user from incurring the consequences of the failure (e.g., document saved
in the event of a sudden and unexpected power failure). Such is the prem-
ise behind the FMEA.

Just as the Shewart cycle represents a systemic way of thinking
about improvement, FMEA represents a systemic way of thinking of
patient safety and medical errors. "Systemic analysis...requires a simul-
taneous imagining of all possible stories...FMEA [does not] refer to a

specific methodology; instead...defines terms of inquiry...'what has failed, what could fail, and how?'.... Given the various possibilities for failure, what are the potential consequences of each?'... [I]n general, a failure is said to occur if a component or a collection of components of a system behaves in a way that is not included in its specified performance criteria" (Senders and Senders 1999, 3.2–3.3).

Although there are several versions of the FMEA (e.g., failure mode analysis and failure mode and criticality analysis), for the purposes of this text, these tools will be discussed under the global term of FMEA. This type of analysis has been used for many years by chemical, structural, mechanical, software, and aerospace engineers. Use of FMEA in healthcare is growing, particularly as JCAHO accreditation standards added a requirement that healthcare facilities identify and conduct at least one FMEA on a high-risk process every year. The FMEA has been used to improve processes and decrease medication errors, reduce adverse events associated with blood administration, improve the safety of IV drug infusions in the pediatric ICU, and reduce patient falls (Cohen 1999; Burgmeier 2002; Apkon et al. 2004; Coles et al. 2005). The FMEA has also been used to improve healthcare facility and product design (Reiling, Knutzen, and Stocklein 2003; Spath 2003).

As with all of the tools described in this chapter, an FMEA is most effective when used in the context of a multidisciplinary team. Once a high-risk process for study has been selected and the team assembled, the line of inquiry goes as follows (Cohen 1999; Spath 2003; Senders and Senders 1999):

* Document the process with a flowchart.
* Anticipate, think of, and describe as many ways as possible in which the process or individual steps in the process could fail.
* List the consequences or effects of the failure.
* Identify the root causes or contributing factors that would lead to the failure.
* On a scale of 1 to 10 (or 1 to 5 for beginners), answer the following questions for each failure:
  a. What is the likelihood of the failure occurring?
  b. How severe could the failure be?
  c. What is the probability that the failure can be detected?
* Multiply the likelihood by the severity by the probability of detection (this is referred to as the criticality score, criticality index, or a risk priority number).
* Using the criticality score, prioritize the failures.
* Improve the process to eliminate the failures.
* Implement the improvements and continue the Shewhart cycle.

Various forms, charts, and matrices to aid in conducting and documenting an FMEA may be found in the web resources section at the end of this chapter.

Root Cause Analysis

The cause-and-effect diagram described earlier in this chapter is one tool used to help document and verify potential root causes of problems. For situations that result in serious or devastating patient outcomes, a deeper inquiry into actual root causes is needed. In the case of a sentinel event, JCAHO requires organizations to conduct a root cause analysis (RCA); implement risk reduction strategies that target the identified root causes; and measure the effectiveness or results of the interventions. JCAHO (2005) defines an RCA as

> a process for identifying the basic or causal factors that underlie variation in performance, including the occurrence or possible occurrence of a sentinel event. A root cause analysis focuses primarily on systems and processes, not individual performance. It progresses from special causes in clinical processes to common causes in organizational processes and identifies potential improvements in processes or systems that would tend to decrease the likelihood of such events in the future, or determines, after analysis, that no such improvement opportunities exist.

This type of RCA is designed to be comprehensive in asking the question "why?" about a wide array of causes, not simply the four categories suggested in the cause-and-effect diagram. Figure 3.14 summarizes the initial questions that should be asked in an RCA.

The companion readings and Internet resources found at the end of the chapter provide a more in-depth explanation and examples of FMEA and RCA.

Conclusion

This chapter provides a general overview of common continuous improvement tools and patient-safety tools. Just as clinical education includes "practice labs" to promote learning while minimizing patient harm, students and practicing managers alike may also learn to use quality tools and approaches in practice labs before they test these tools in ways that affect their organization, employees, and, ultimately, patients.

The exercises in this chapter may be viewed as such a lab for managers as they practice an improvement process and an error investigation. The last two tools presented—FMEA and RCA—begin to bridge traditional quality tools with contemporary tools incorporating a systems approach. Section II introduces quality management from a systems approach. Chapter 4 explores concepts of systems thinking and dynamic complexity as expressed in healthcare organizations.

- Briefly summarize the circumstances surrounding the occurrence, including the patient outcome (e.g., death, loss of function).
- Who participated in the analysis?
- When did the event occur?
- What area/service was impacted?
- Include the full variety of services impacted by the event.
- What are the steps in the process, as designed?
- What human factors were relevant to the event?
- How could equipment performance affect the outcome?
- What controllable factors directly affected the outcome?
- Where there uncontrollable external factors?
- What other areas or services are impacted?
- To what degree is staff properly qualified and currently competent for their responsibilities?
- How did actual staffing compare with ideal levels?
- What are the plans for dealing with contingencies that would reduce effective staffing levels?
- How has staff performance in the relevant processes been assessed? When was this last performed?
- How can orientation and in-service training be improved?
- To what degree is all information available when needed?
- To what degree is communication among participants adequate?
- To what degree was the physical environment appropriate for the processes being carried out?
- What emergency and failure mode responses have been planned and tested?
- To what degree is the culture conducive to risk identification and reduction?
- Did the overall culture of the facility encourage or welcome change, suggestions, and warnings from staff regarding risky situations or problematic areas?
- Does management establish methods to identify areas of risk or access employee suggestions for change? Are changes implemented in a timely manner?
- What are the barriers to communication of potential risk factors?
- To what degree is the prevention of adverse outcomes communicated as a high priority?
- What can be done to protect against the effects of uncontrollable factors?
- Was a literature search done?

FIGURE 3.14
JCAHO's Tool for Conducting a Root Cause Analysis: An Excerpt

Source: © Joint Commission on Accreditation of Healthcare Organizations, 2005. Reprinted with permission.

Companion Readings

McKee, J. (ed.). 2005. *Root Cause Analysis in Health Care: Tools and Techniques,*
  3rd edition. Oakbrook Terrace, IL: Joint Commission Resources, Inc.
Scholtes, P. R., B. L. Joiner, and B. J. Streibel. 2003. *The Team Handbook,*
  3rd edition. Madison, WI: Oriel Inc.
Senders, J. W. 2004. "FMEA and RCA: The Mantras of Modern Risk
  Management." *Quality and Safety in Healthcare* 13: 249–50.
Smith, I. J. (ed.). 2005. *Failure Mode and Effects Analysis in Health Care:*
  Proactive Risk Reduction, 2nd edition. Oakbrook Terrace, IL: Joint
  Commission Resources, Inc.

Web Resources

Improvement Tools

American Society of Quality: www.asq.org/learn-about-quality/quality-tools.html
Institute for Healthcare Improvement: www.ihi.org/IHI/Topics
  /Improvement/ImprovementMethods/Tools

Patient Expectations

Eight Dimensions of Patient-Centered Care (text and flash movie):
  http://nrcpicker.com/Default.aspx?DN=112,22,2,1,Documents

Patient Safety

Institute for Safe Medication Practices: www.ismp.org
Advances in Patient Safety: From Research to Implementation, Volumes 1-4:
  www.ahrq.gov/qual/advances/

Patient Safety Tools: Failure Mode and Effects Analysis

Veteran's Administration National Center for Patient Safety:
  www.patientsafety.gov/SafetyTopics.html
American Society of Quality: www.asq.org/learn-about-quality
  /process-analysis-tools/overview/fmea.html
Joint Commission International Center for Patient Safety:
  www.jcipatientsafety.org/show.asp?durki=10364

Patient Safety Tools: Root Cause Analysis

Veteran's Administration National Center for Patient Safety:
  www.patientsafety.gov/rca.html
Joint Commission International Center for Patient Safety (Preparing for an RCA):
  www.jcipatientsafety.org/show.asp?durki=10365&site=180&return=9808
Joint Commission International Center for Patient Safety (Sentinel Event
  Resources): www.jcipatientsafety.org/show.asp?durki=9368

References

Apkon, M., J. Leonard, L. Probst, and R. Vitale. 2004. "Design of a Safer Approach to Intravenous Drug Infusions: Failure Mode Effects Analysis." *Quality and Safety in Healthcare* 13: 265–71.

Bingham, T. 2005. Excerpt from an unpublished document.

Burgmeier, J. 2002. "Failure Mode and Effect Analysis: An Application in Reducing Risk in Blood Transfusion." *The Joint Commission Journal on Quality Improvement* 28 (6): 331–39.

Cohen, M. R. 1999. "One Hospital's Method of Applying Failure Mode and Effects Analysis." In *Medication Errors*, edited by M. R. Cohen, 4.1–4.4. Washington, DC: American Pharmaceutical Association.

Coles, G., B. Fuller, K. Kordquist, and A. Kongslie. 2005. "Using Failure Mode Effects and Criticality Analysis for High-Risk Processes at Three Community Hospitals." *The Joint Commission Journal on Quality and Patient Safety* 31 (3): 132–40.

Critical Thinking Community. 2005. "Defining Critical Thinking." [Online information; retrieved 10/8/05.] www.criticalthinking.org/aboutCT /definingCT.shtml.

Facione, P. A., N. C. Facione, C. A. F. Giancarlo, and S. W. Blohm. 2005. "Teaching for Thinking." [Online information: retrieved 5/5/06.] www.insightassessment.com/pdf_files/CT_Teaching_tips.pdf.

Gerteis, M., S. Edgman-Levitan, J. Daley, and T. L. Delbanco (eds.). 1993. *Through the Patient's Eyes: Understanding and Promoting Patient-Centered Care.* San Francisco: Jossey-Bass.

Institute for Clinical Systems Improvement. 2003. "About ICSI." [Online information; retrieved 06/28/02.] www.icsi.org/about/.

———. 2005. "Diagnosis and Treatment of ST Elevated Acute Myocardial Infarction." [Online information.] www.icsi.org/.

Institute for Healthcare Improvement. 2003. "Breakthrough Series Collaboratives." [Online information; retrieved 06/06/02.] www.ihi.org/collaboratives/breakthroughseries/.

Joint Commission on Accreditation of Healthcare Organizations (JCAHO). 2005. "Tool to Assist Organizations in the Completion of the Framework for Conducting a Root Cause Analysis." [Online information; retrieved 5/5/06.] www.jcipatientsafety.org/show. asp?durki=9754&site=165&return=9368.

Juran, J. M. 1989. *Juran on Leadership for Quality: An Executive Handbook.* New York: The Free Press.

Kelly, D. L. 1998. "Reframing Beliefs About Work and Change Processes in Redesigning Laboratory Services." *Joint Commission Journal on Quality Improvement* 24 (9): 154–67.

Langley, G. J., K. M. Nolan, T. W. Nolan, C. L. Norman, and L. P. Provost. 1996. *The Improvement Guide: A Practical Approach to Enhancing Organizational Performance.* San Francisco: Jossey-Bass.

NRC+Picker. 2005. "Eight Dimensions of Patient Care." [Online information; retrieved 12/20/05.] nrcpicker.com /default.aspx?DN=112,22,2,1,Documents.

Pougnet, T. 1996. Presentation at LDS Hospital, Salt Lake City, Utah, May 20–23.

Reiling, J. G., B. L. Knutzen, and M. Stocklein. 2003. "FMEA—The Cure for Medical Errors." *Quality Progress* 36 (8): 67–71.

Scholtes, P. R., B. L. Joiner, and. B. J. Streibel. 2003. *The Team Handbook, 3rd edition*. Madison, WI: Oriel Inc.

Senders, J. W., and S. J. Senders. 1999. "Failure Mode and Effects Analysis in Medicine." In *Medication Errors*, edited by M. R. Cohen, 3.1–3.8. Washington, DC: American Pharmaceutical Association.

Spath, P. L. 2003. "Using Failure Mode and Effects Analysis to Improve Patient Safety." *Association of Operating Room Nurses Journal* 78: 16–37.

Walton, M. 1986. *The Deming Management Method*. New York: The Putnam Publishing Group.

Exercise 1

Objective: To practice quality improvement tools by applying them to an improvement effort in an ambulatory care setting.

Instructions

1. Read the following case study.
2. Follow the instructions at the end of the case.

Case Study

Background
You have just been brought in to manage a portfolio of several specialty clinics in a large multiphysician group practice in an academic medical center. The clinics reside in a multiclinic facility that houses primary care and specialty practices as well as a satellite laboratory and radiology and pharmacy services. The practice provides the following centralized services for each of its clinics: registration, payer interface (e.g., authorization), and billing. The CEO of the practice has asked you to initially devote your attention to Clinic X to improve its efficiency and patient satisfaction.

Access Process
A primary care physician (or member of the office staff), patient, or family member calls the receptionist at Clinic X to request an appointment. If the receptionist is in the middle of helping a patient in person, the caller is asked to hold. The receptionist then asks the caller, "How may I help you?" If the caller is requesting an appointment within the next month, the appointment date and time is made and given verbally to the caller. If the caller asks additional questions, the receptionist provides answers. The caller is then given

the toll-free preregistration phone number and asked to preregister before the date of the scheduled appointment. If the requested appointment is beyond a 30-day period, the caller's name and address are put in a "future file" because physician availability is given only one month in advance. Every month, the receptionist reviews the future file and schedules an appointment for each person on the list, and a confirmation is automatically mailed to the caller.

When a patient preregisters, the financial office is automatically notified and performs the necessary insurance checks and authorizations for the appropriate insurance plan. If the patient does not preregister, when the patient arrives in the clinic on the day of the appointment and checks in with the specialty clinic receptionist, he or she is asked to first go to the central registration area to register. If there is an obvious problem with authorization, it is corrected before the patient returns to the specialty clinic waiting room.

The receptionist has determined that the best way to not inconvenience the caller is to keep him or her on the phone for as short an amount of time as possible. The receptionist also expresses frustration with the fact that there are too many things to do at once.

Physician's Point of View

The physician thinks too much of his or her time is spent on paperwork and chasing down authorizations. The physician senses that appointments are always running behind and that patients are frustrated, no matter how nice he or she is to them.

Patients' Point of View

Patients are frustrated when asked to wait in a long line to register, which makes them late for their appointment, and when future file appointments are scheduled without their input. As a result of this latter factor, and work or childcare conflicts, patients often do not show up for these scheduled appointments.

Office Nurse's Point of View

The office nurse feels that he or she is playing catch up all day long and explaining delays. The office nurse also wishes there was more time for teaching.

Billing Office's Point of View

The billing office thinks some care is given that is not reimbursed because of inaccurate or incomplete insurance or demographic information or that care is denied authorization after the fact.

Data

On the NRC+Picker website you find the following patient expectations/dimensions of care for adults and children in their outpatient experiences with a hospital or clinic outpatient appointment:

- Respect for patients' values, preferences, and expressed needs
- Coordination and integration of care
- Information and education
- Physical comfort

- Emotional support and alleviation of fear and anxiety
- Involvement of family and friends
- Transition and continuity
- Access to care

The clinics have just begun to monitor performance data, and you have one quarter's worth of data for the clinic:

Overall satisfaction with visit	82%
Staff is courteous and helpful	90%
Waiting room time is less than 15 minutes	64%
Examination room waiting time is less than 15 minutes	63%
Patient no-show rate	20%
Patient cancellation rate	11%
Provider cancellation rate	10%
Preregistration rate	16%
Average number of patient visits per day	16
Range of patient visits per day	10–23

Instructions

1. Completely read all of the instructions.
2. Decide which problem you want to focus on as your first priority— the goal for your improvement team.
3. Identify the team members that you would want to participate in this effort and what fundamental knowledge they should bring to the process.
4. Document the current process using a process flowchart.
5. Identify your customers and their expectations.
6. Prioritize opportunities to improve by doing the following:
   a. Complete an RCA using a fishbone diagram with the following categories: people (patients), people (staff/employees), policies and procedures, and plant (facilities/equipment);
   b. Describe how you would collect data about how often the root causes contribute to the problem to determine where your greatest opportunity for improvement would be; and
   c. Design a Pareto chart from the data given in the table above (you may also use hypothetical data to design your Pareto chart).
7. Review the following change concepts (Langley et al. 1996), and identify the ones that may apply to your process:
   - Eliminate waste (e.g., things that are not used, intermediaries, unnecessary duplication)
   - Improve workflow (e.g., minimize handoffs, move steps in the process closer together, find and remove bottlenecks, do tasks in parallel, adjust to high and low volumes)
   - Manage time (e.g., reduce set-up time and waiting time)

- Manage variation (create standard processes where appropriate)
- Design systems to avoid mistakes (use reminders)

8. Improve the process and document the improved process with a process flowchart or workflow diagram.
9. Decide what you will measure and briefly describe how you would collect the data.
10. You have completed the "Plan" phase of the Shewhart cycle. Describe briefly how you would complete the rest of the PDCA cycle.
11. Save your answers to each part of this exercise. This will become the documentation of your improvement effort.

Exercise 2

Objective: To practice an RCA.

Instructions

1. Read the following case study.
2. Follow the instructions at the end of the case.

Case Study

The letter in this case study is adapted with permission from Trina Bingham, master's in nursing student at Duke University School of Nursing.

You are the risk manager of a tertiary-care hospital and have just received the following letter from a patient who was recently discharged from your facility.

> Dear Risk Manager,
> Last month, I had surgery at your hospital. I was supposed to have a short, laparoscopic surgery with a discharge by lunch, but it turned into an open surgery with complications. This led to a 4-day hospital stay and discharge with a Foley catheter. Overall, my hospital stay was OK, but I had a situation when the call bell was broken. It was during the night, and I was alone. I needed pain meds. I kept ringing the call bell and no one answered. I used my phone to call the switchboard and no one answered. I didn't want to yell. My IV began beeping (to be honest I kinked the tubing to make it beep), but no one came with that noise either. Eventually the certified nursing assistant (CNA) came to routinely check my vitals and she got a nurse for me. They switched call bells, but apparently there was an electrical problem, and the call bell couldn't be fixed until the next day when maintenance was working. The CNA told me to "holler if I needed

anything" as she walked out closing the door. I was so mad, but by this time, the IV pain med was working and I was dosing off. I reported the situation again on day shift and even spoke to the director of nursing and the quality assurance manager. Upon discharge, I included this dangerous and unethical situation on my patient satisfaction survey. But I have to wonder when these data are combined with all the other data if the situation looks insignificant. For me, it worked out OK. All I needed was pain medicine, but what if I had needed help for something more serious? Depending on the layout of satisfaction and quality of care survey results; this situation could look very minor. For all I know, my dissatisfaction was under the heading "dissatisfied with room."

I am writing to you because I have not heard from the director of nursing or the quality assurance manager about what they have done to fix the problems. I believe it is important that you hear my complaint so hopefully other patients will not have to go through the terrible experience that I did.

To fix the problems described in this patient's letter, you realize you must first understand the root causes of the problems. Although this situation did not result in a sentinel event, you realize that it could have and decide to conduct an RCA. Brainstorm possible responses to the RCA questions in Figure 3.14.

THE SYSTEMS APPROACH

4

A SYSTEMS PERSPECTIVE OF QUALITY MANAGEMENT

Objectives

- To introduce the concept of systems thinking
- To introduce the concept of dynamic complexity
- To provide examples that illustrate dynamic complexity in healthcare
- To explore the implications of dynamic complexity for healthcare managers

As people accumulate years of experience in the healthcare field, they begin to see the recurring problems—sometimes within an individual organization, sometimes across the entire industry. Problems thought to be solved by one manager may come back at a later time for a different manager. The CEO of a large hospital may eliminate the case management department to meet necessary budget cuts for the year; three years later, the new CEO of the same hospital may create a case-management department to address numerous problems with the patient discharge process. Consider the following situation (Georgopoulos and Mann 1962, 549–51):

> The hospital faces a number of problems concerning the nursing staff . . . one major problem is...attracting and retaining a sufficient professional nursing staff, especially non-supervisory nursing staff... [T]he problem lies in the fact that the number of professional nurses being trained in nursing schools is much too low to meet an ever increasing demand for professional nurses by hospitals and other sources...[B]eing understaffed, hospitals often assign to the professional nurse a rather heavy workload that is not seen as normal or reasonable by many nurses... [A]nother important problem...involves the composition of the total nursing staff, the question of optimum balance in the proportions of staff members who are registered nurses, practical nurses, and aides.

Although this situation may appear to address a manager's current challenges with nursing shortages, the above excerpt was taken from the book *The Community General Hospital*, which was published in 1962! During the more-than-40 years since that book was written, healthcare organizations seem to have made little headway in issues related to workforce planning and management. Nursing shortages, for example, have appeared and disappeared in waves in the 1960s, 1970s, 1980s, early 1990s, and again in the early years of the twenty-first century.

Why do budget problems and nursing shortages remain nagging issues for healthcare managers? The reasons lie in the complex nature of healthcare, healthcare organizations, and the healthcare industry. By "complex" we mean the presence of a large number of variables that interact with each other in innumerable ways. In addition to the presence of many variables, healthcare and healthcare systems are characterized by situations in which "cause and effect are not close in time and space and obvious interventions do not produce expected outcomes" (Senge 1990, 71). This characteristic represents another type of complexity, known as dynamic complexity. Although an intervention may appear to be the obvious solution at the time, if it does not alter the fundamental behavior of the system that is causing the problem, the solutions are only temporary. As seen in the nursing shortage example, although interventions may offer temporary relief, the problems resurface again and again.

In healthcare, as in other industries, "systems thinking is needed more than ever because we are being overwhelmed with complexity" (Senge 1990, 69). This chapter introduces a systems perspective of quality management that is based on the concepts of systems thinking and dynamic complexity.

Systems Thinking

In Chapter 1, a variety of perspectives surrounding the term "quality" are discussed. Likewise, the term "system" brings with it numerous connotations and perceptions. Depending on the source, system may be defined in a variety of ways in healthcare organizations or in healthcare. In this book, system refers to a collection of parts that interact with each other to form an interdependent whole (Kauffman 1980; Scott 1998).

Although a system reflects the whole, "systems thinking is a discipline for seeing wholes. It is a framework for seeing interrelationships, rather than things, for seeing patterns of change rather than static 'snapshots'" (Senge 1990, 68). Systems thinking acknowledges the large number of parts in a system, the infinite number of ways in which the parts interact, and the nature of the interactions. Systems thinking implies that one must read between the elements of a system to understand how they are connected.

Dynamic Complexity

Several system characteristics contribute to the presence of dynamic complexity (Sterman 2000). Five characteristics, predominant in healthcare and healthcare organizations, are described in this section: change, trade-offs, history dependency, tight coupling, and nonlinearity.

Change

Systems are dynamic—that is, changing. Change occurs at different rates and scales within and among systems, especially in healthcare. Consider three levels of dynamic complexity in healthcare. First, the human body changes continuously. This means that key inputs (patients with a clinical problem) to and outputs (patients' status after clinical intervention) of healthcare systems represent moving targets. Second, the organizational contexts in which healthcare and healthcare delivery are carried out are dynamic in nature. Employees move in and out of organizations, research provides an ongoing stream of new clinical interventions, and technological advances offer new clinical and management approaches. Third, the communities and political environments in which we live and in which healthcare organizations operate change—that is, the environment changes with economic cycles, political ideologies, and election cycles.

From the day a person is born to the day he dies, that person is in a constant state of change, growing and developing physiologically and emotionally. No two human systems are exactly alike or precisely predictable in their response to a medical intervention. As a result, functions that may seem straightforward in other industries, such as product standardization, become more difficult for healthcare managers. For example, many organizations use the practice of pharmacy benefits management (PBM), a hospital formulary using a standardized list of drug names and brands to reduce medication expenses. However, when the dynamic nature of patient physiology is introduced, the manager recognizes that in addition to the question, "What are the set of drug names and brands that will be most cost-effective?" she also needs to ask, "How should the approved drugs be selected, and what are the consequences to patients?"

Implications for Healthcare Managers

To aid in grasping the subtle but important nuances involved in individualizing treatment plans, the metaphor of trying on a pair of blue jeans may be used. People have their own favorite brand of blue jeans that "fit," even though another brand may be advertised as having a similar size and style. Likewise, despite similar biochemical structures, certain medications may work better for one person than for another because of the individual's genetic makeup. The PBM essentially dictates to doctors that the patient may buy only slim-cut size 10 jeans and not relaxed-fit size 10 jeans (Kelly and Pestotnik 1998; Weisman 2005).

An alternative approach to PBM that takes into account the dynamic nature of patient physiology as well as the need to reduce costs is seen in the computer-assisted management program for antibiotics and other anti-infective agents. With this tool, the computer gathers the extensive and complex information about the patient (e.g., vital signs, laboratory and other diagnostic information), the medication (e.g., dose, frequency, route, contraindications), the clinical evidence (e.g., relevant published studies, use in other similar patients), and the costs of optional therapies. The software program continually updates the most current version of all the necessary decision elements (patient, medical evidence, costs, and safety considerations) and presents the information to care providers at the point of service so that they may make timely decisions about the most appropriate, safe, and cost-effective intervention (Evans et al. 1998; Mullett et al. 2001).

Trade-Offs

The need to understand the nature of trade-offs may seem unnecessary for managers taught to weigh pros versus cons or opportunities versus risks as they consider organizational decision options. Trade-offs may be seen as an accepted attribute of management. However, an understanding of dynamic complexity can shed light on the system consequences of local management trade-off decisions. Trade-offs are seen in dynamically complex systems because "time delays in feedback channels mean the long-run response of a system to an intervention is often different from its short-run response. High leverage policies often cause worse-before-better behavior, while low leverage policies often generate transitory improvement before the problem grows worse" (Sterman 2000, 22).

Implications for Healthcare Managers

A classic example of a low-leverage policy, as defined above, was published in the *New England Journal of Medicine* (Fitzgerald, Moore, and Dittus 1988). Although a 1988 publication may be viewed as dated, the lessons for managers in this article are even more relevant today than when the study was published.

The advent of prospective payment systems in 1983 drove many hospitals to reduce costs by decreasing patient length of stay. This article examined the impact of these practices on quality of care for elderly patients with hip fractures. As Table 4.1 summarizes, the variables studied included length of stay, number of physical therapy sessions, functional status measured by the distance in feet that patients could walk, percentage of patients discharged to nursing homes, and percentage of patients still in nursing homes one year after discharge. If a manager in this case defined the healthcare system as "the orthopedic department/unit" or the hospital administrator defined the healthcare system as "this hospital," the intervention chosen to reduce healthcare system costs appeared to be appropriate. In this article, the decision and subsequent interventions to reduce length of stay appeared to be successful; mean hospital stay declined from 21.9 to 12.6 days. In addition, "neither in-hospital mortality nor one-year mortality changed significantly" (Fitzgerald, Moore, and Dittus 1988, 1392). Based on these criteria—length of hospital stay, hospital mortality,

	Before	**After**
Length of stay	21.9 days	12.6 days
Physical therapy sessions	7.6	6.3
Functional status (measured by distance in feet walked)	93	38
Percentage of patients discharged to nursing homes	38%	60%
Percentage of patients still in nursing homes one year after discharge	9%	33%

TABLE 4.1
Impact of Low-Leverage Policy: Reducing Hospital Costs by Reducing Hospital Length of Stay

Source: Adapted with permission from Table 2 in "The Care of Elderly Patients With Hip Fracture. Changes Since Implementation of the Prospective Payment System" by J. F. Fitzgerald, P. S. Moore, and R. S. Dittus, in the *New England Journal of Medicine* 319 (21): 1394. Copyright © 1988 Massachusetts Medical Society. All rights reserved.

and one-year mortality—a manager could be confident that this was a successful cost-reduction strategy.

However, if one defines the healthcare system as including not only the acute phase of care (e.g., orthopedic unit, hospital) but also the downstream providers (e.g., rehabilitation and long-term care) and takes into account how the relationships among all providers influence patient outcomes, the longer-term behavior of the system can be observed. The short-term intervention of reducing length of stay, and in turn reducing physical therapy sessions and functional status, also led to an increase in patients discharged from the hospital directly to nursing homes. The authors concluded that the result was a shift in "much of the rehabilitation burden to nursing homes" (Fitzgerald, Moore, and Dittus 1988, 1392), and they observed a subsequent increase in the percentage of patients remaining in nursing homes one year after hospital discharge. Overall costs related to the consumption of healthcare resources for the care of these patients actually increased.

To this finding, a manager may respond, "But my responsibility is only my unit/hospital." From a systems perspective, the acute care manager is responsible not simply for the acute care unit or hospital but also for the impact those local decisions have on the rest of the system of which the manager's component is a part. This does not mean that the manager of the orthopedic department or the hospital administrator should not strive to reduce hospital costs. It does mean, however, that managers, financial officers, CEOs, and policymakers should be aware of how decisions made and implemented within their domains of responsibility affect other parts of the healthcare system, both positively and negatively. When a negative impact to another part of the system is anticipated, the manager should be proactive in the short term to help minimize the negative effects and preserve positive patient outcomes. In the case presented in this article, a proactive intervention would have been to ensure that nursing homes had adequate rehabilitation capacity before reducing hospital length of stay.

Other common trade-off challenges for healthcare managers surround the differences between expense and investment decisions within organizations and departments. The long-term effect of a manager's short-term decision may not be felt by another component in the system (e.g., nursing home, patient) as in the previous example, but perhaps it will surface at a certain point in the future within the manager's own department or organization. For example, does the manager sacrifice capital improvements to fund traveling nurses in the short term? Do managers reduce staff education dollars to reduce current expenses? Although choosing traveling nurses and reducing staff development activities may meet the short-term need to reduce expenses, these efforts fall into the category of low-leverage policies because the problems of facility aging, staff shortages, and the need for a competent workforce will surely be faced by the manager in the future. Without an appreciation of system consequences, one manager may be rewarded for the short-term "success" with a promotion, while his successor inherits the longer-term problem.

In the PBM example, the organization may be willing to trade off the rare adverse medication event for dollar savings realized from product standardization. However, this type of micro (patient level)/macro (organizational level) trade-off that allows for patient status to be potentially compromised may unintentionally contribute to polarization and conflict between clinicians and managers.

History Dependency

Systems are history dependent. In other words, what has happened in the past influences what is occurring in the present. Some actions are reversible, but many actions are not.

Implications for Healthcare Managers

Once again, this characteristic may be seen in both the patient and the organization. For example, even though a person stopped smoking at the age of 40, the effects of 25 years of a two-pack-per-day habit will dictate this person's health and care requirements for the rest of his or her life. Individual patient histories influence how a manager interprets performance data. Adjusting clinical outcomes for patient acuity (e.g., presence of comorbidities) or adjusting overall organizational acuity takes into account the patient as a dynamic system and is an essential system tool for data analysis in healthcare (Iezzoni 1997).

Another example of this characteristic is illustrated by how a healthcare organization's past decision to pursue or not pursue electronic information systems affects its ability to meet current information demands and reporting requirements. The ability of the healthcare industry to manage information and report performance pales in comparison to that of other industries such as financial services. Consider the following perspective: "If you go to the doctor, the doctor is recording your visit in vegetable pigment on crushed wood fibers. This is literally a medieval method of data storage and retrieval. I ask you, how would you react if you went to a bank and asked for money and someone opened up a big, old ledger and blew it off and said, 'Oh, let's see, how much do you have?'" (Smith 2002).

The manager must realize not only how past events have shaped current events but also how past decision-making strategies and directions may influence her ability to successfully achieve current and future goals. Using the information systems example, if the organization has historically rewarded managers for quarterly or annual financial performance, a large capital investment today for a future financial gain may be very difficult to sell given the reward and decision-making history of the organization.

Tight Coupling

A system is characterized as tightly coupled when "the parts exhibit relatively time-dependent, invariant, and inflexible connections with little slack" (Scott 1998, 351) and when "the actors in the system interact strongly with one another" (Sterman 2000, 22).

Implications for Healthcare Managers

Following routine procedure at the airport, a traveler gives his airline boarding pass and photo identification to the security check-point agent. The agent returns them, explaining that the boarding pass and identification do not match and that the traveler must return to the ticket counter to have the discrepancy corrected. The ticket agent generates a new boarding pass for the nonstop flight and apologizes for the inconvenience. Upon arrival at the destination, the traveler discovers that his checked suitcase is missing. Unknown to the traveler, the ticket agent's computer generates the boarding pass and luggage tag concurrently. Although the agent correctly fixed the boarding pass, the process had already been set in motion for the suitcase to travel under the original incorrect name to the incorrect destination.

As this example illustrates, the consequences of tight coupling occur whether workers operating within the system are aware of them or not. Depending on their work histories and backgrounds, students and managers may or may not have experienced a work setting that is tightly coupled. Typically, knowledge work is not considered tightly coupled, while certain production and mechanical processes are considered as such. Although healthcare delivery is typically thought of as a service, many work processes within such an organization are actually closer in nature to production processes than to service processes, causing the organization to potentially be considered tightly coupled. Healthcare managers who have never actually worked in a tightly coupled system or environment must learn about and gain an appreciation for this system characteristic to be effective in their roles.

A "code" for a cardiac arrest is an example of a healthcare process that is very tightly coupled. Each person on the team carries out his or her respective steps in this emergency process in a specific order, and many steps depend on a previous step. An IV line must be in place before certain medications can be administered. The patient's age and weight determine the exact dosage of medication to be given; inaccurate calculations can have disastrous results.

Specific work settings and environments in a hospital are also considered tightly coupled, including processes, procedures, and staff in operating rooms and ICUs. Even the concept of continuum of care implies a certain degree of coupling among the patient, the primary care physician, acute care, long-term care, and home care.

Seemingly benign processes, when viewed from one point of view (i.e., in terms of cost or acuity), may actually be considered tightly coupled when viewed another way (i.e., in terms of the number of interactions within the system required to successfully and safely complete the process). Studies by the Healthcare Advisory Board have shown that a typical x-ray procedure may take up to 40 steps, involve 15 to 20 employees, and require up to 148 minutes from start to finish (The Advisory Board Company 1992). This example alone begs healthcare managers to include work simplification and job design—techniques that have been used in other industries for years—in all improvement efforts (Hackman and Oldham 1980).

Organizations in industries outside of healthcare that are most commonly identified as tightly coupled include nuclear power plants and aircraft carriers. These work environments pose unique organizational and management challenges. As the study of human error and human factors is becoming more visible and accepted within healthcare practice, managers may increasingly take lessons from what are referred to as high-reliability organizations and bring those lessons back to healthcare settings (Reason 1990, 1997; Roberts 1990; Weick and Sutcliffe 2001).

Nonlinearity

The term "nonlinear" as it refers to a system characteristic means that the "effect is rarely proportional to the cause" (Sterman 2000, 22) and that, because the parts in the system may interact in numerous ways, these interactions may follow "unexpected sequences that are not visible or not immediately comprehensible (Scott 1998, 351).

Implications for Healthcare Managers

A nurse just starting the afternoon shift is the object of an outburst of anger from a patient's family. The nurse relates the encounter to a colleague at the nurse's station: "All I did was say, 'Hello'!" This situation may bring to mind the old cliché "the straw that broke the camel's back." In fact, this cliché is an accurate description of the encounter.

The patient and her family had accumulated a sequence of unsatisfactory experiences during the hospital stay, so all it took was one more encounter to trigger their anger. The afternoon nurse, although this was the first time he had met the family, was the last in a series of interactions between the patient and the healthcare system that caused this family to use the nurse as a target of their frustration. Now, if the patient complains to the manager about this nurse, what can the manager do? If the manager does not have an appreciation for the nonlinear nature of systems, she may be tempted to discipline the nurse. However, if the manager does have an appreciation for the nonlinear nature of systems, she may try to recreate with the family the sequence of events, although each was relatively harmless when considered individually, that when linked together with the family's situation contributed to an extremely dissatisfying experience. From this investigation, the manager may identify areas that can be improved to enhance the patient's overall experience with the care-delivery process.

Another example of the nonlinear nature of systems may be seen in strategies used to reduce personnel expense in healthcare organizations. Because personnel expenses make up such a large percentage of operating budgets, changing the staff mix—that is, reducing the number of professional staff (e.g., registered nurses, medical technologists, pharmacists) and increasing the proportion of assistive personnel (e.g., nurses' aides, laboratory assistants, pharmacy technicians)—is a common cost-cutting intervention. When this intervention is studied from a systems perspective, however, the resulting sequences of activities and their interrelationships are more readily seen. The unplanned consequences of this cost-cutting strategy in one organization included an increase in the overall employee turnover rate because of the high turnover among the entry-level, assistive personnel group. Because this cost-cutting strategy was used by managers across different types of professions and departments, the stress and cost of continuously recruiting, hiring, and training new employees more than offset the savings hoped for from lowering the average hourly wage. When viewed from one department's point of view, the cost-reduction strategy may appear to be reasonable; however, when the compounding effect of this cost-cutting strategy is viewed across the entire organization, the strategy designed to reduce costs is actually undermining the organization's ability to do so (Kelly 1999).

The nonlinear characteristics of the larger healthcare system can be seen when other consequences of this particular cost-cutting strategy are examined: "[B]ecause some local schools decide their enrollments based on the current number of job openings in a particular field, hospital staffing decisions made today can affect the number of qualified job applicants available in four to five years. For example, from 1994 to 1996, local hospitals aggressively reduced positions for registered nurses. Applications for enrollment at a local nursing school dropped by 41 percent during the same time period" (Kelly 1999, 10).

This effect was not only seen with nurses but also with medical technologists and radiology technicians. This realization, gained through a systems perspective of the organization's cost-cutting strategies, prompted the organization to reevaluate its staffing practices and succession planning and to begin aggressively coordinating with local schools to proactively prepare for future staff shortages. This organization began addressing staff shortages a full three years before the staff shortages in healthcare resurfaced as a widespread concern in 2001 (Kelly 1999; Knox, Irving, and Gharrity 2001).

Conclusion

This chapter introduces the concepts of systems thinking and dynamic complexity as they apply to healthcare and healthcare organizations. Chapter 5 expands on the concept of systems thinking by introducing several systems models that managers may use to better understand the relationships among variables within their own organizations. Understanding these system relationships provides insight into the subtle, but powerful, factors that contribute to the organization's ability to progress along the quality continuum. The exercise at the end of this chapter provides readers with an opportunity to practice identifying dynamic complexity in a patient care experience.

Companion Readings

Coutou, D. L. 2003. "Sense and Reliability: A Conversation with Celebrated Psychologist Karl E. Weick." *Harvard Business Review* 81 (4): 84–90.

Senge, P. M. 1990. "The Leader's New Work: Building Learning Organizations." *Sloan Management Review* (Fall): 149–65.

Weick, K. E., and K. M. Sutcliffe. 2001. *Managing the Unexpected: Assuring High Performance in an Age of Complexity*, 1–23. San Francisco: Jossey-Bass.

References

The Advisory Board Company. 1992. *Re-Engineering the Hospital: CEO Primer on Bottlenecks, Excess Cost and Lost Revenue*. Washington, DC: The Advisory Board Company.

Evans, R. S., S. L. Pestotnik, D. C. Classen, T. P. Clemmer, L. K. Weaver, J. F. Orme, J. F. Lloyd, and J. P. Burke. 1998. "A Computer-Assisted Management Program for Antibiotics and Other Antiinfective Agents." *New England Journal of Medicine* 338 (4): 232–38.

Fitzgerald, J. F., P. S. Moore, and R. S. Dittus. 1988. "The Care of Elderly Patients with Hip Fracture. Changes Since Implementation of the Prospective Payment System." *New England Journal of Medicine* 319 (21): 1392–97.

Georgopoulos, B. S., and F. C. Mann. 1962. *The Community General Hospital.* New York: The MacMillan Company.

Hackman, J. R., and G. R. Oldham. 1980. *Work Redesign.* Reading, MA: Addison-Wesley Publishing Company.

Iezzoni, L. I. (ed.). 1997. *Risk Adjustment for Measuring Healthcare Outcomes, 2nd edition.* Chicago: Health Administration Press.

Kauffman, D. R. 1980. *Systems One: An Introduction to Systems Thinking.* Minneapolis, MN: Future Systems, Inc.

Kelly, D. L. 1999. "Systems Thinking: A Tool for Organizational Diagnosis in Healthcare." In *Making It Happen: Stories from Inside the New Workplace,* compiled from The Systems Thinker Newsletter, 1989–97. Waltham, MA: Pegasus Communications, Inc.

Kelly, D. L., and S. L. Pestotnik. 1998. "Using Causal Loop Diagrams to Facilitate Double Loop Learning in the Healthcare Delivery Setting." Unpublished manuscript.

Knox, S., J. A. Irving, and J. Gharrity. 2001. "The Nursing Shortage—It's Back!" *JONAS Healthcare, Law, Ethics and Regulation* 4 (2): 31.

Mullett, C. J., R. S. Evans, J. C. Christensen, and J. M. Dean. 2001. "Development and Impact of a Computerized Antiinfective Decision Support Program." *Pediatrics* 108 (4): e75.

Reason, J. 1990. *Human Error.* Cambridge, UK: Cambridge University Press.

———. 1997. *Managing the Risks of Organizational Accidents.* Hampshire, UK: Ashgate Publishing Limited.

Roberts, K. 1990. "Some Characteristics of One Type of High Reliability Organization." *Organizational Science* 1: 160–76.

Scott, W. R. 1998. *Organizations: Rational, Natural and Open Systems, 4th edition.* Upper Saddle River, NJ: Prentice Hall.

Senge, P. M. 1990. *The Fifth Discipline: The Art and Practice of the Learning Organization.* New York: Doubleday Currency.

Smith, M. 2002. "Quality Measurement in Healthcare: The Role of Public Reporting." University of North Carolina at Chapel Hill, School of Public Health Program on Health Outcomes, 2002 Spring Seminar Series, March 27.

Sterman, J. D. 2000. *Business Dynamics: Systems Thinking and Modeling for a Complex World.* Boston: Irwin McGraw-Hill.

Weick, K. E., and K. M. Sutcliffe. 2001. *Managing the Unexpected: Assuring High Performance in an Age of Complexity.* San Francisco: Jossey-Bass.

Weisman, J. 2005. "Drugmakers Win Exemption in House Budget-Cutting Bill." *Washington Post,* November 30, A08.

Exercise

Objective: To practice identifying dynamic complexity in a patient care experience.

Instructions

1. Read the case study.
2. Review the system characteristics that contribute to dynamic complexity:
   - Change
   - Trade-offs
   - History dependency
   - Tight coupling
   - Nonlinearity
3. Explain how these system characteristics are expressed in the case study.

Case Study

This case is adapted from Kelly, D. L., and S. L. Pestotnik. 1998. "Using Causal Loop Diagrams to Facilitate Double Loop Learning in the Healthcare Delivery Setting." Unpublished manuscript.

Mrs. B was a 66-year-old widow living on a fixed income. She had been diagnosed with high blood pressure and osteoporosis. Her private doctor knew her well. When he selected the medication with which to treat her high blood pressure, he took into account her age, the fact that she had osteoporosis, and other issues. He chose a drug that had proven beneficial for patients like Mrs. B and that had minimum side effects. Mrs. B did well on the medication for ten years. Her insurance covered the cost of her medication, except for a small out-of-pocket copayment.

The last time Mrs. B went to her local pharmacy to refill her prescription, the pharmacist informed her that her insurance company had contracted with a PBM company. (The role of a PBM company is to perform a variety of cost-cutting services for health-insurance plans. One of these services is to decide which drugs an insurance company will pay for; the PBM company's preferred-product list is known as a formulary.) If Mrs. B wanted to continue to take the same medication, it would cost her five times her usual copayment. She was quite disturbed because she could not afford this price increase and did not fully understand her insurance company's new policy. The pharmacist offered to call Mrs. B's doctor, explain the situation, and ask him whether he would change her prescription to the PBM-preferred brand. When the physician was contacted, he was not aware of the PBM company's action and was not completely familiar with the preferred product. The pharmacist discussed Mrs. B's predicament with the physician and described the financial consequences of her continuing to receive her original prescription. After this discussion with the pharmacist, the physician concluded that his only option was to approve the switch, which he did.

Mrs. B began taking the new brand of high blood pressure medicine. One week after starting on the new drug, she developed a persistent cough that aggravated her osteoporosis and caused her rib pain. When the cough and pain continued for another week, Mrs. B began to take over-the-counter medicines for the pain. She unknowingly opened herself to having a reaction between her blood pressure medication and the pain medication: orthostatic hypotension (lightheadedness when rising from a lying to an upright position). One morning on her way to the bathroom, she fainted, fell, and broke her hip. She was admitted to the hospital for surgery, where she developed a urinary tract infection. The infection spread to her repaired hip, which resulted in a bloodstream infection that eventually led to her death.

SYSTEMS MODELS FOR HEALTHCARE MANAGERS

Objectives

- To describe four systems models for healthcare managers
- To discuss selected lessons for healthcare managers from each model

Just as a road map provides a picture of how places are connected in a geographic area, systems models can provide a picture for managers of how elements may be connected within and to an organization. Numerous models provide healthcare managers with a picture of the organizational system in which they work. Different models may resonate with different managers depending on their work settings, backgrounds, and individual preferences. The model that the manager selects is less important than how he or she uses it to begin recognizing, understanding, and anticipating how the parts of the systems interact as a whole.

The most basic system may be characterized by three elements: input(s), a conversion process, and output(s). These elements are demonstrated visually in the simple diagram below:

Input(s) ➡ Conversion process ➡ Output(s)

In a health services organization, examples of inputs are patients, personnel, supplies, equipment, facilities, and capital. Examples of a conversion process are diagnostic processes, clinical treatments, operational activities, and business management functions. Examples of outputs are a patient's health status and an organization's business performance.

Traditional quality efforts may be thought of in terms of managing the elements of the system. Examples of ways to control the quality of personnel inputs include licensure requirements, continuing education, and performance appraisals. Examples of ways to control the quality of technology inputs like drug therapies include clinical trials and U.S. Food and Drug Administration approval. Examples of ways to control the quality of a conversion process include clinical guidelines, process improvement, or work simplification. Controlling the quality of the inputs and conversion processes is intended to improve the quality of the outputs, such as patient clinical and functional status, satisfaction with services, cost effectiveness, employee behaviors, and organizational culture.

FIGURE 5.1
Quality
Management
System

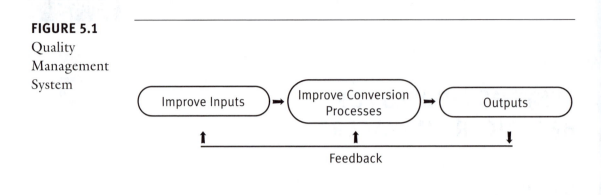

Adding a feedback loop changes this basic system to a more dynamic one and, in turn, leads to a more mature approach to quality efforts. Feedback about the quality of the outputs guides efforts to improve the quality of the inputs and the conversion processes. Continuous feedback promotes continuous improvement (see Figure 5.1). While similar to Donabedian's three quality measures, which are discussed in Chapter 1 (structure, process, outcomes), the focus here includes the entire organization, not simply those clinical or medical elements of the system.

In Chapter 4, systems thinking is defined as "a discipline for seeing wholes. It is a framework for seeing interrelationships, rather than things, for seeing patterns of change rather that static 'snapshots'" (Senge 1990). Improving the quality of the parts and understanding and improving the quality of the relationships between the parts lead managers to the most mature—or systems thinking—approach to quality management in their organizations.

Four models are presented in this chapter: the three core process model, the Baldrige National Quality Program (BNQP) Healthcare Criteria for Performance Excellence, the systems model of organizational accidents, and the socioecological framework.

Three Core Process Model

The three core process model shown in Figure 5.2 represents a "horizontal" view of a healthcare delivery organization (Kelly et al. 1997; Ostroff and Smith 1992); all processes in the organization (represented by the arrows) should operate in an aligned fashion toward improving performance. The model starts on the right of the figure by defining desired results. A balanced set of patient outcomes, taken from the clinical value compass (Nelson et al. 1996), is used to describe the desired results in clinical outcomes, functional status, satisfaction against need, and cost. This model describes organizational culture and employee behaviors as outcomes or outputs of the organizational processes.

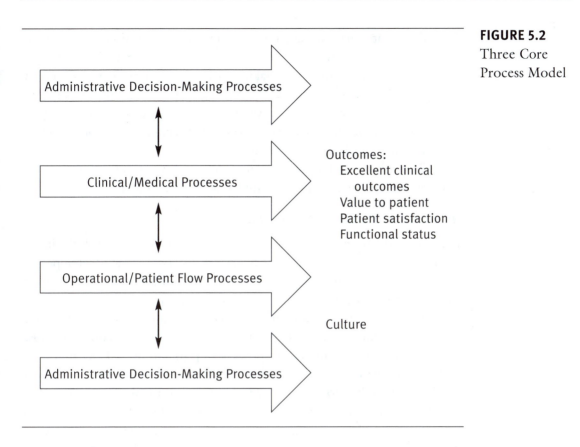

FIGURE 5.2
Three Core
Process Model

Administrative Decision-Making Processes

Clinical/Medical Processes

Outcomes:
  Excellent clinical
    outcomes
  Value to patient
  Patient satisfaction
  Functional status

Operational/Patient Flow Processes

Culture

Administrative Decision-Making Processes

According to the three core process model, although many processes take place in a healthcare delivery organization, they may be grouped into three core categories: (1) clinical processes, (2) operational or patient flow processes, and (3) administrative processes.

Clinical/medical processes are the fundamental reasons patients seek the services of a healthcare organization—that is, to address some clinical need that may include processes related to diagnosis, treatment, prevention, and palliative care. Clinical/medical processes include those under the domain of physicians as well as those under the domain of nonphysicians. The processes may be medical (e.g., physician), such as surgery; may be related to improving the individual's functional status, such as physical therapy; may be related to daily care that the individual or family is unable to carry out without help, such as nursing care after an accident; or may be related to receiving special medication or respiratory treatments, such as oxygen and IV medication for a person with pneumonia.

Operational/patient flow processes are those that enable a patient to access the clinical processes during his or her visit or course of stay. This core category includes processes that involve the following: registering and admitting the patient to the facility, administering diagnostic tests, determining what unit the patient goes to and when the patient is transferred or discharged, ensuring that the patient receives meals or medications at the appropriate time, and preparing the patient and family members for discharge.

Administrative decision-making processes occupy two positions in the figure, above and below the other two core processes. In this way, the model illustrates how administrative processes influence the overall organization. These processes include decision making, communication, resource allocation, and performance evaluation.

The arrows linking the three core processes reflect the interdependence of the processes in leading to desired outcomes.

Lessons for Healthcare Managers

The three core process model teaches managers several lessons. First, the interdependent relationships between the three core processes suggest that improvement in any one of these processes has the potential to increase the value of the service provided; however, the concurrent targeting of these core processes provides a synergy that can accelerate the achievement of improved outcomes. "An efficient clinical process supported by an inefficient operational process, or vice versa, is still an inefficient process.... [I]n addition, if...changes are made independent of clinician involvement, the likelihood of implementation is reduced. It is therefore necessary to have decision-making processes that actively engage clinicians in change efforts" (Kelly et al. 1997, 127–28).

For example, in one ambulatory surgery unit, the patient postoperative length of stay—from the time the patient leaves the operating room to the time the patient is discharged—was found to be longer than in similar ambulatory surgery units. An improvement effort was initiated to address the postoperative care process so that the discharge process could be improved and, in turn, the length of stay could be reduced. As the improvement effort progressed, the team realized that anesthesia practices were affecting their ability to achieve better results. If patients were being heavily sedated in the operating room and were slow to wake up as a result, then the gains from improving the postoperative process could not be fully realized. Likewise, if the physicians implemented a new clinical protocol for anesthesia and pain management but patients still had to wait for the nurses to discharge them, gains from improving the anesthesia process could not be fully realized. Recognizing the interdependence of these two processes and targeting both the discharge process and the anesthesia protocol for improvement allowed the benefits of both improvement efforts to be achieved. Furthermore, if the administrative processes did not permit employees to be scheduled away from work so they could be involved in the quality efforts, neither of the improvements could take place at all.

Second, the three core process model helps promote a patient-focused orientation by visibly aligning processes and improvement efforts toward the needs of the patient. The conceptual view of operations and administration is always in the context of how the patient moves through the entire system to access a clinical process. For example, a seemingly simple super-visory decision such as scheduling lunch breaks took on new meaning for one emergency department when the decision was viewed in conjunction with patient flow. Although scheduling staff lunch breaks at noon seemed reasonable, this practice created unnecessary patient delays and bottlenecks in the patient care processes because patient visits for follow-up care typi-cally increased during the hours of 11:00 a.m. to 1:00 p.m. If the depart-ment's focus was the patients, then staff should be present when patients needed them. As a result, the break policy was revised so that staff breaks occurred before and after—rather than during—busy patient times.

Third, the model reinforces the different yet necessary and interde-pendent contributions that each core process and the providers/implementers of those processes provide to patient care and organizational outcomes. This way, collaboration among the entire care team can be promoted, as one administrator told a group of physicians: "I am not going to tell you how to practice medicine. However, it is important that I know your needs so that you may deliver quality care, and you need to know the constraints I am under to provide you with what you need. The best decisions will come by working and planning together."

Fourth, when the administrative role is viewed as a process rather than a function or a structure, all of the tools used to improve other types of processes may also be applied to administrative processes to help man-agers improve their own effectiveness. If one of the desired outcomes is patient satisfaction, the administrative decision-making processes must include mechanisms to collect, analyze, report, communicate, and evalu-ate patient satisfaction data on a regular basis.

The Baldrige National Quality Program Healthcare Criteria for Performance Excellence

The BNQP Healthcare Criteria for Performance Excellence provide the most contemporary framework for organizational effectiveness as described in Chapter 1 (Dean and Bowen 1994). For readers who desire a more in-depth explanation, a complete version of these criteria and examples of how health services organizations address the criteria may be found on the Baldrige website (see the web resources at the end of the chapter).

Figure 5.3 illustrates the essential elements in the model and the links between these elements. The following passage explains how to read and inter-pret the figure (National Institute of Standards and Technology 2006, 6):

> Your organizational profile (top of figure) sets the context for the
> way your organization operates. Your environment, key working
> relationships, and strategic challenges serve as an overarching
> guide for your organizational performance management system.

The system operations are composed of the six Baldrige categories in the center of the figure that define your operations and the results you can achieve. Leadership; Strategic Planning; and Focus on Patients, Other Customers, and Markets represent the leadership triad. These categories are placed together to emphasize the importance of a leadership focus on strategy and patients and other customers. Senior leaders set your organizational direction and seek future opportunities for your organization.

Human Resource Focus, Process Management, and Results represent the results triad. Your organization's staff and its key processes accomplish the work of the organization that yields your performance results.

All actions point toward Results—a composite of healthcare, patient and other customer, and market, financial, and internal operational performance results, including human resource, governance, and social responsibility results.

The horizontal arrow in the center of the framework links the leadership triad to the results triad, a linkage critical to organizational success. Furthermore, the arrow indicates the central relationship between Leadership and Results. The two-headed arrow indicates the importance of feedback in an effective performance management system.

Measurement, Analysis, and Knowledge Management are critical to the effective management of your organization and to a fact-based, knowledge-driven system for improving health care and operational performance. Measurement, analysis, and knowledge management serve as a foundation for the performance management system.

Lessons for Healthcare Managers

Managers may take several lessons from the BNQP systems model. First, the model describes the essential elements for organizational effectiveness (represented by the seven boxes in the model) and how they are related. The model recognizes the unique circumstances in which different organizations operate and encourages managers to base decisions, strategies, and interventions on the organizational profile. The overarching nature of the organizational profile promotes ongoing consideration of external influences such as environmental, regulatory, or market demands.

When viewed in light of the BNQP model, one can see that the principles of total quality, (customer focus, continuous improvement, and teamwork) described in Chapter 2, address some required elements (focus on

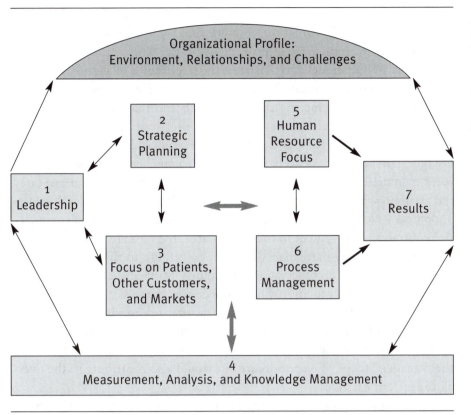

FIGURE 5.3

Baldrige
Healthcare
Criteria for
Performance
Excellence
Framework

Source: National Institute of Standards and Technology. 2006. "Baldrige National Quality Program Healthcare Criteria for Performance Excellence." [Online information; retrieved 1/2/06]. www. baldrige.gov/Criteria.htm.

patients, other customers, and markets; process management; and human resource focus) but not all of the required elements. The BNQP model suggests that quality management in a healthcare organization requires managers to focus attention not only on the three principles of total quality but also on the way leadership, strategic planning, measurement, analysis and knowledge management, and a broader focus on human resources contribute to achieving the desired organizational performance results.

For example, managers who use this model understand the link between the elements of process management and human resource needs. Before implementing a process improvement, managers would ask themselves, "What needs to happen to ensure that the staff will succeed at implementing the new process?" As a result, managers may need to overstaff when a new process is initially implemented to give employees some leeway as they learn the new process or their new roles. Adapting to something new takes time, and by planning ahead, the manager may be able to negotiate for the short-term budget or productivity variances required for the transition period. An understanding of the BNQP model helps managers realize that their role in process improvement also includes ensuring that employees have the information, training, and tools they need so that they may successfully implement improvements in the work setting.

The BNQP model also illustrates the importance of alignment within the organization. This means that the activities within each box in the model are directed toward achieving the same results and that organizational and management choices are consistent with the organization's mission, vision, values, strategic direction, and patient and stakeholder requirements. For example, one healthcare delivery system offers comprehensive quality improvement training for its managers. Each manager is expected to design and carry out an improvement project as a requirement of the training, so each selects a topic on which to focus his improvement project. Although each manager demonstrates improvement in the chosen area, the collective improvements of all of the training participants may not contribute to the overall organizational objectives. This observation is illustrated by one manager who devoted much time and effort to improving a service area that was eliminated by the organization the following year. Another healthcare organization offering a similar type of training for managers used senior leaders to help the managers select improvement topics that would not only provide benefit within the managers' scope of responsibility but would also contribute to the overall organizational goals.

This model emphasizes the importance of alignment of data, analysis, and performance indicators. Managers using the BNQP model would choose performance indicators in a systematic way. When designing their performance measurement system and selecting performance indicators, managers may consistently ask themselves the following series of questions (National Institute of Standards and Technology 2006):

- What are the key determinants of success for our setting of care?
- Who are our patients and stakeholders, and what are their requirements?
- How do these determinants and requirements guide decisions about our organizational goals?
- Are these goals consistent with the mission, vision, and values of the organization?
- What approach(es) will we use to meet our goals?
- What is the desired impact for selecting this particular approach?
- What performance indicators will allow us to measure the desired impact?
- How often should each of these indicators be reviewed, and by whom?
- What data collection, analysis, and reporting capabilities are necessary to deliver the performance indicators as determined?

Finally, the BNQP model provides the manager with a vehicle for initiating and continuing discussions about performance excellence within the organization.

Systems Model of Organizational Accidents

James Reason's systems model of organizational accidents is intended to explain how medical errors may occur in health services organizations. This model not only takes into account the relationships between elements in the system, but it also integrates the characteristics of dynamic complexity described in the previous chapter.

To understand Reason's model, one must first understand the definitions and assumptions upon which it is based. An *error* is defined as "all those occasions in which a planned sequence of mental or physical activities fails to achieve its intended outcome" (Reason 1990, 9). Errors may be further categorized as *judgment errors* (improper selection of an objective or plan of action), *execution errors* (proper plan carried out improperly), *errors of omission* (something that should be done is not done), and *errors of commission* (something that should not be done is done) (Reason 1990; Institute of Medicine 1999).

Active errors are those committed by frontline workers, and the results are seen immediately (Reason 1990; 1997). For example, a restaurant-server trainee picks up a hot plate by mistake, quickly lets it go, and watches the plate and its contents crash to the kitchen floor. *Latent errors*, on the other hand, occur in the upper levels of the organization. The error may lie dormant for days or years until a particular combination of circumstances allows the latent error to become an adverse event (Reason 1990; 1997). For example, a restaurant customer, thinking she has bitten a seed of some sort in the salad, removes a metal button from her mouth instead. Angry at her subsequent chipped tooth, she demands compensation from the restaurant's owner and threatens to report the incident to the local health department. Upon investigating the incident, the owner discovers that since the restaurant changed uniform vendors several months previously, there have been numerous reports from staff that the quality of the new uniform deteriorates quickly after multiple washings. The button in question had probably loosened in the laundry and gone unnoticed by the chef when it fell off during routine meal preparation.

Finally, Reason's model assumes there are usually a collection of defenses that act as buffers or safeguards to prevent a hazardous situation from becoming an adverse event, just as a thick oven mitt would prevent the restaurant worker from dropping the hot dish in the example above. The collection of defenses in an organization may be thought of as several slices of Swiss cheese lined up next to each other. The holes in the slices of cheese represent the latent and active errors present in the organization. Even though an error may be present (i.e., a hole in one slice), it does not result in an adverse event or accident because there are organizational defenses to stop it from continuing (i.e., the next slice). For example, in hospitals, it is becoming common practice for pharmacists to review physicians' medication orders before dispensing the medication to the patient care unit. A physician may inadvertently write an incorrect dosage; however, when the pharmacist picks up the mistake and clarifies the order with the physician (organizational defense), a medical error is prevented.

Figure 5.4 illustrates the slices of Swiss cheese (or collection of defenses). The figure shows that under certain circumstances, the interplay between latent errors, local conditions, and active errors causes the holes in the cheese to align just right so that a sequence of events may pass through all the holes and result in an adverse event.

Lessons for Healthcare Managers

Administrative and management professionals play key roles in medical errors as they are the source of latent errors in organizations (Reason 1997, 10).

> Latent conditions are to technical organizations what resident pathogens are to the human body. Like pathogens, latent conditions—such as poor design, gaps in supervision, undetected manufacturing or maintenance failures, unworkable procedures, clumsy automation, shortfalls in training, less than adequate tools and equipment—may be present for years before they combine with local circumstances and active failures to penetrate the system's many layers of defenses. They arise from strategic and other top-level decisions made by governments, regulators, manufacturers, designers and organizational managers. The impact of these decisions spreads throughout the organization, shaping a distinctive corporate culture and creating error-producing factors within the individual workplaces.... Latent conditions are an inevitable part of organizational life. Nor are they necessarily the products of bad decisions, although they may well be. Resources, for example, are rarely distributed equally between organization's various departments. The original decision on how to allocate them may have been based on sound...arguments, but all such inequities create quality, reliability, or safety problems for someone, somewhere in the system at some later point.

Frontline employees or those in direct contact with patients serve as both the last layer of defense to prevent an error as well as the last layer where a defense may break down. While the results of a sequence of events leading to the medical error or adverse event are seen at the point of patient contact, the causes may be found throughout all levels of the organization. Reason describes the role of the frontline staff as "rather than being the main instigators of an accident...tend to be the inheritors of system defects created by poor design, incorrect installation, faulty maintenance, and bad management decisions. Their part is usually that of adding the final

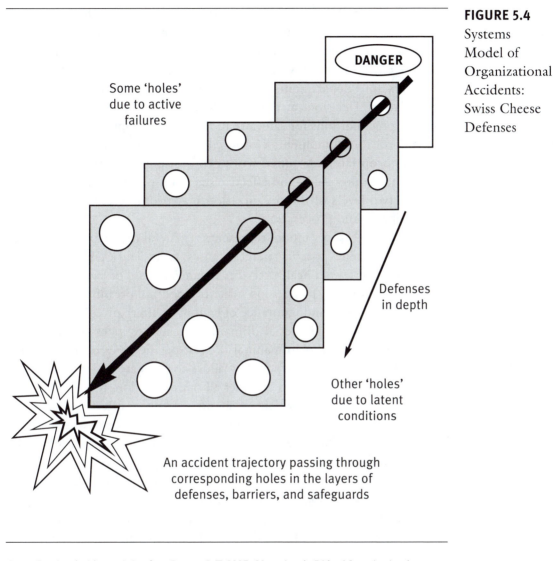

FIGURE 5.4

Systems Model of Organizational Accidents: Swiss Cheese Defenses

Source: Reprinted with permission from Reason, J. T. 1997. *Managing the Risks of Organizational Accidents.* Hampshire, United Kingdom: Ashgate Publishing Limited.

garnish to a lethal brew whose ingredients have already been long in the cooking" (Reason 1990, 173).

Chapter 2 discusses the role of organizational design and the principles of quality management. Likewise, Reason's model emphasizes the role of organizational design in medical errors. Latent errors may occur at the level of senior leaders, who design organizational goals and priorities and determine how human, financial, and capital resources are allocated. Latent errors may also occur at the level of frontline managers who translate and implement senior-level goals and priorities within their own scope of responsibilities. Frontline management includes those responsible for departments that provide direct care or patient service (e.g., professional, allied health, technical), departments that maintain and support the environment in which care is provided and the tools used by care providers, and departments that support the business functions of the organization. Decisions at these two levels of the organization, in turn, support preconditions for safe care in the form of appropriate, functioning, and reliable equipment; a knowledgeable, skilled, and trained workforce; appropriately designed work processes, communication mechanisms, and staffing plans; and effective supervision. Alternatively, decisions at these two levels of the organization may promote error-prone work environments and processes.

While Reason's model represents a general organizational model, Hofmann examines specific sources, causes, types, and examples of latent management errors in health services organizations. For example, "inadequate preparation of/by decision maker(s), political pressure, flawed decision-maker process, and ignorance of legitimate alternatives" are causes of errors within the managerial domain of health services organizations (Hofmann 2005, 10). Hofmann also cites specific types of management errors. Errors of omission include "failure to delegate and hold subordinates accountable; failure to consider all options; failure to balance power interests; and, failure to anticipate significant factors affecting decisions" (Hofmann 2005, 11.) Errors of commission include "permitting decisions to be made without adequate analysis; choosing political, not business solutions; withholding negative information from individuals with the right to know; and making economic decisions that harm clinical care and outcomes" (Hofmann 2005, 11). An understanding of Reason's model emphasizes the imperative for managers' knowledge, skill, and abilities to complement their clinical and technical counterparts in the organization.

Socioecological Framework

The socioecological framework is a systems perspective on promoting health that comes from the field of health behavior and health education. This field uses and reflects theory from many disciplines, including psychology, sociology, political science, education, cultural anthropology, biostatistics, epidemiology, health policy, and business administration. The socioecological framework, in turn, provides an integrated and multidisciplinary systems perspective on health and health behaviors (Reed 2001).

The socioecological framework is shown in Figure 5.5. Reading the figure top to bottom illustrates the four levels of determinants of health behavior: individual, organization, community, and population (Reed 2001; Stokols 1992). Reading the figure left to right illustrates that for each of

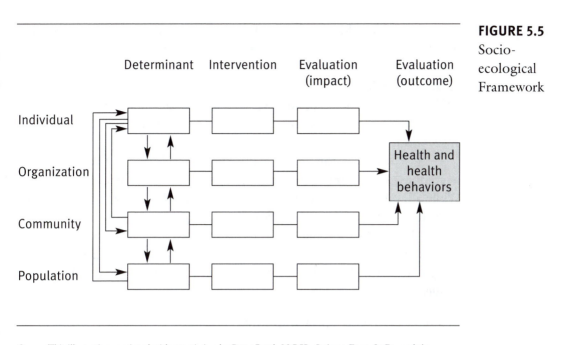

FIGURE 5.5

Socio-ecological Framework

Source: This illustration reprinted with permission by Peter Reed, M.P.H., JoAnne Earp, Sc.D., and the instructors of HBHE 131, *Introduction to Social Behavior in Public Health,* Department of Health Behavior and Health Education, University of North Carolina at Chapel Hill, School of Public Health, 2001.

these levels of determinants, specific interventions may be implemented and their impact evaluated. For example, the model may be used to better understand smoking behavior.

Individual determinants of smoking behavior include a person's knowledge of associated health risks and the smoking behavior of family and friends. Individual interventions to reduce smoking behaviors may include smoking-cessation classes and pharmacotherapy (e.g., nicotine patches). The impact is measured by whether the person stops smoking or does not start in the first place.

Organization determinants of smoking behavior include policies regarding smoking in the workplace and the availability of smoking-cessation classes as an employee health benefit. Prohibiting smoking, offering limited access to onsite smoking areas, and reimbursing employees for smoking-cessation classes are interventions targeted at the organizational level. The proportion of employees who smoke or the "quit rate" is the organizational evaluation measure.

Community determinants of smoking behavior include social norms and beliefs. For example, smoking may be linked to social status and acceptance. Because of the history of tobacco farming in the southeastern United States, smoking has also been associated with the community's economic livelihood. Redefining social norms and recruiting nontobacco economic opportunities would be considered community-level interventions. Impact may be measured in terms of community smoking rates.

Population determinants of smoking behavior include regulations regarding smoking in public places. Interventions such as no-smoking airline flights, no-smoking buildings, or a "sin tax" on cigarettes are examples of population-level interventions. The effect may be measured by compliance with regulations and population smoking rates.

In the figure, the arrows between the levels indicate the interconnectedness of the determinants, interventions, and impact at all levels. While a level-specific intervention may be effective, recognizing the relationships between the levels creates a synergy to enhance desired outcomes. Using the example above about smoking, one can understand the limited impact of enrolling a person in a smoking-cessation class when he is surrounded by smokers in the family, in the workplace, and in public venues.

Lessons for Healthcare Managers

The major lesson from this model for healthcare managers is that it provides a more expansive view of the nature of health in general and of healthcare delivery specifically. In doing so, the model offers a larger context from which to understand interventions designed to improve the quality and safety of services provided by healthcare organizations and, in turn, understand complementary and/or competing interventions within and between levels. For example, without an understanding of issues at the state and policy levels related to topics such as disclosure; privilege; contract and tort law; and industry regulations, such as JCAHO requirements, practitioners may inadvertently be placed at legal risk when asked by managers to participate in efforts to identify, report, analyze, and reduce errors in the clinical practice environment (Liang 1999, 2000; Liang and Cullen 1999). Even though a healthcare manager may not be responsible for such policy decisions, her awareness of the interaction of the levels in the socioecological framework can provide the impetus and direction for establishing community partnerships and evaluating intended and unintended consequences of quality interventions within her own organization.

In 2001, the Institute of Medicine recommended that "the changes needed to realize a substantial improvement in health care involve the health care system as a whole" (Institute of Medicine 2001, 20). This recommendation implies understanding not only how organizations work as systems but also how the multiple players and layers involved in the healthcare industry are interrelated. The socioecological framework can help managers understand the increasing activity on the part of professional societies; regulatory agencies; and local, state, and federal governments to improve the quality and safety of healthcare.

Three Core Process Model	Baldrige National Quality Program	Systems Model of Organizational Accidents	Socioecological Framework
Encourages concurrent improvement of interdependent processes	Shows how the components of performance excellence are related	Explains administrators and managers as sources of latent errors	Broadens and expands the manager's view
Aligns processes around patient needs	Recognizes the context in which the organization operates	Describes frontline consequences of system errors	Addresses community and policy influences on health outcomes
Values all provider/ employee groups	Promotes alignment of all activities within the organization	Emphasizes importance of management competence	
Views administrative role as a process rather than a function	Promotes alignment of performance indicators		
	Enhances communication around performance excellence		

TABLE 5.1

Systems Models: Lessons for Managers

Conclusion

This chapter presents four different systems models for managers. Table 5.1 summarizes key lessons for managers in each of these models. Whichever model the manager chooses to use, the common benefit of using systems models is that they encourage the manager to do the following:

- broaden his perspective to see his own work environment, department, and organization within a larger context;
- better understand the interconnectedness and relationships between various components within an organization that contribute to performance results;
- realize that results are achieved by design, that design is a choice, and that to achieve better results, he must improve the quality of his choices; and
- appreciate the role of community- and population-level initiatives targeted toward improving quality and safety in healthcare.

The exercises at the end of this chapter provide an opportunity to use the systems models to better understand how organizational relationships influence quality. Chapter 6 explores the role of public and private policy relative to healthcare quality.

Companion Readings

Baldrige National Quality Program. 2006. "Healthcare Criteria for Performance Excellence." [Online information; retrieved 1/2/06.] www.baldrige.gov /Criteria.htm.

Reason, J. 2000. "Human Error: Models and Management." *Western Journal of Medicine* 172: 393–96.

Web Resources

Federal Quality Program

Baldrige National Quality Program: www.baldrige.nist.gov/index.html

Baldrige Healthcare Criteria for Performance Excellence: www.baldrige.gov/Criteria.htm

Baldrige National Quality Award Winners (Healthcare): Organizational profiles, contact information, and award application summaries: www.baldrige.nist.gov/Contacts_Profiles.htm

> 2005 Bronson Methodist Hospital
> 2004 Robert Wood Johnson University Hospital, Hamilton
> 2003 Saint Luke's Hospital of Kansas City, and Baptist Hospital, Inc.
> 2002 SSM Health Care

Additional Resources

Anesthesia Patient Safety Foundation: www.apsf.org/

American Nurses Association National Center for Nursing Quality: www.nursingworld.org/quality/

National Database of Nursing Quality Indicators: www.nursingquality.org

Kaiser Family Foundation: www.kaiseredu.org/

References

Dean, J. W., and D. E. Bowen. 1994. "Management Theory and Total Quality: Improving Research and Practice Through Theory Development." *Academy of Management Review* 19 (2): 392–418.

Gibson, R., and J. P. Singh. 2003. *Wall of Silence: The Untold Story of the Medical Mistakes That Kill and Injure Millions of Americans.* Washington, DC: LifeLine Press.

Hofmann, P. B. 2005. "Acknowledging and Examining Management Mistakes." In *Management Mistakes in Healthcare: Identification, Correction and*

Prevention, edited by P. B. Hofmann and F. Perry, 3–27. Cambridge, UK: Cambridge University Press.

Institute of Medicine. 1999. *To Err Is Human: Building a Safer Health System*, edited by L. T. Kohn, J. M. Corrigan, and M. S. Donaldson. Washington, DC: National Academies Press.

———. 2001. *Crossing the Quality Chasm: A New Health System for the 21st Century*. Washington, DC: National Academies Press.

Kelly, D. L., S. L. Pestotnik, M. C. Coons, and J. W. Lelis. 1997. "Reengineering a Surgical Service Line: Focusing on Core Process Improvement." *American Journal of Medical Quality* 12 (2): 120–29.

Liang, B. A. 1999. "Error in Medicine: Legal Impediments to U.S. Reform." *Journal of Health Politics, Policy and Law* 24 (1): 27–58.

———. 2000. "Creating Problems as Part of the 'Solution': The JCAHO Sentinel Event Policy, Legal Issues and Patient Safety." *Journal of Health Law* 33 (2): 263–85.

Liang, B. A., and D. J. Cullen. 1999. "The Legal System and Patient Safety: Charting a Divergent Course: The Relationship Between Malpractice Litigation and Human Errors." *Anesthesiology* 91 (3): 609–11.

National Institute of Standards and Technology. 2006. "Baldrige National Quality Program Healthcare Criteria for Performance Excellence." [Online information; retrieved 1/2/06.] www.baldrige.gov/Criteria.htm.

Nelson, E. C., J. J. Mohr, P. B. Batalden, and S. K. Plume. 1996. "Improving Healthcare, Part 1: The Clinical Value Compass." *Joint Commission Journal on Quality Improvement* 22 (4): 243–58.

Ostroff, F., and D. Smith. 1992. "The Horizontal Corporation: It's About Managing Across, Not Up and Down." *The McKinsey Quarterly* 1992 (1): 148–68.

Reason, J. 1990. *Human Error*. Cambridge, UK: Cambridge University Press.

———. 1997. *Managing the Risks of Organizational Accidents*. Hampshire, UK: Ashgate Publishing Company.

Reed, P. 2001. "Introduction to Social Behavior in Public Health." Course lecture at the Department of Health Behavior and Health Education, University of North Carolina at Chapel Hill, School of Public Health.

Senge, P. M. 1990. The Fifth Discipline: *The Art and Practice of the Learning Organization*. New York: Doubleday Currency.

Stokols, D. 1992. "Establishing and Maintaining Healthy Environments: Toward a Social Ecology of Health Promotion." *American Psychologist* 47 (1): 6–22.

Exercise 1

Objective: To practice identifying relationships within systems.

Instructions

1. Review the four systems models presented in this chapter:
    *   Three core process model
    *   BNQP Healthcare Criteria for Performance Excellence

- Systems model of organizational accidents
- Socioecological framework
2. Choose one that you can best relate to at this time.
3. Review your responses to the Chapter 1 exercise. Look at both your excellent quality experience and your poor quality experience, paying particular attention to how you described the manager's role or influence.
4. Now, think about those experiences from the perspective of the systems model you chose in question 2. Describe any additional understanding of the experience that you may have when viewing it from a systems perspective, then write your responses in a table similar to the one below.

Systems Model Worksheet

	Manager's role/influence	Additional understanding by viewing through systems perspective
Excellent Quality Experience		
Poor Quality Experience		

Exercise 2

Objective: To practice identifying different types of errors.

Instructions

Consider the following scenario.

> In Florida, Clara, an active ninety-four-year-old great-grandmother who still worked as a hospital volunteer two days a week, was admitted to the hospital for a bowel obstruction. She and her family, along with nurses from the hospital, said that there were too few nurses to check her during the night when her eldest son went home to sleep for a couple of hours. Clara called the nurses to help her use the bathroom but when no one came, she climbed over the bed railing. Still groggy from surgery twenty hours earlier, Clara fell to the floor and broke her left hip. She died two days later during surgery to repair the hip fracture. "It was just too much for her," said her grandson. "For want of one nurse, she died" (Gibson and Singh 2003, 101).

Using the information provided in this chapter, brainstorm and list possible factors that may have contributed to this patient's death. Use the following categories as a guide:

- Latent failures at the level of senior decision makers
- Latent failures at the level of frontline management
- Latent failures at the level of workplace preconditions
- Specific circumstances surrounding this event
- Active errors associated with this event

EXPANDING THE BOUNDARIES OF THE SYSTEM: THE ROLE OF POLICY

Objectives

- To review concepts related to health policy
- To explore the role of public and private policies on healthcare quality

Policies that control water, air, and food quality and, in turn, their respective impacts on preventing disease in populations are fundamental to public health practice. Public policy also plays a role in promoting the quality of healthcare delivery services. Physicians, nurses, nurse practitioners, pharmacists, and other care providers require licenses to practice their professions and are guided by the statutes and rules outlined in the professional practice acts and occupational licensing bodies of their respective states. A physician's office may display evidence of professional credentials such as diplomas and board certification. Likewise, one will find evidence of the organizational credentials in the form of business licenses or accreditations posted visibly for customers, patients, and visitors. The ramped sidewalk to the front door of a health facility and tiny Braille numbers on the elevator buttons are design features influenced by the Americans with Disabilities Act. Sprinklers in the ceilings, signs labeled as "fire exit," and special doors designed to close automatically fulfill building codes and fire safety requirements. Inappropriate or excessive radiation exposure to patients and healthcare personnel during diagnostic exams is prevented through meeting Occupational Safety and Health Administration requirements. The safety and efficacy of medications are investigated, tested, and approved by the U.S. Food and Drug Administration before release for patient use.

While funding, payment, and access legislation, such as Medicare and Medicaid, may be the most visible or well-known topics of healthcare policy, the examples above illustrate how public policy also plays an integral role in ensuring the quality of many other aspects of healthcare services. Historically, policy initiatives have targeted the quality of the *structural elements* of the healthcare delivery system, such as people, physical facilities, equipment, and drugs. For many years, the public health infrastructure on the state, national, and international levels has collected and reported aggregate outcome measures, such as infant mortality rates and life expectancy, and aggregate process measures, such as immunization rates. Current targets of policy initiatives for healthcare quality are organization-specific, provider-specific, population-specific, and disease-specific processes and outcomes.

Chapter 5 introduces four systems models. Two of these models—the socioecological framework and the BNQP Healthcare Criteria for Performance Excellence—address the role of external influences that shape how health services organizations operate. Chapter 2 discusses the expanding influence of the business community in defining quality requirements for health services organizations. This chapter addresses the increasingly important role of public and private policies on healthcare quality. First, a brief overview of health policy concepts is presented, followed by a description of the federal healthcare-quality reporting initiatives, JCAHO's redesigned accreditation approach, and how these initiatives are based on and incorporate a systems approach.

Health Policy: An Overview

The U.S. government serves the following generic purposes: "to provide for those who cannot provide for themselves, to supply social and public goods, to regulate the market, and to instill trust and accountability" (Longest 2002, 48). To accomplish these purposes, the government uses *public policy* or "authoritative decisions made in the legislative, executive, or judicial branches of government that are intended to direct or influence the actions, behaviors, or decisions of others" (Longest 2002, 11). Complementing public policy is *private sector policy*, which guides governance and operations within a specific organization or as established by private organizations for the purpose of industry oversight (Longest 2002).

Regulatory policies are used to promote societal objectives in situations in which private markets do not function properly according to competitive market rules. These policies are designed to control economic forces, such as market entry, price, and quality, as well as to promote social aims, such as ensuring workplace safety and preventing spread of communicable disease (Longest 2002). *Allocative policies* are "designed to provide net benefits to some distinct group or class of individuals or organizations, at the expense of others, to ensure that public objectives are met" (Longest 2002, 33). For example, taxes provide pools of dollars that are redistributed to fund public goods and services such as roads and law enforcement. *Health policies* are defined as policies that "pertain to health or influence the pursuit of health" (Longest 2002, 11). Health policies are crafted to influence health determinants, which in turn influence health. The Healthy People 2010 model, shown in Figure 6.1, illustrates the relationship among health policies, health determinants, and health.

Health-quality policy may be thought of as a subset within health policy. Government policies promote healthcare quality in a variety of ways,

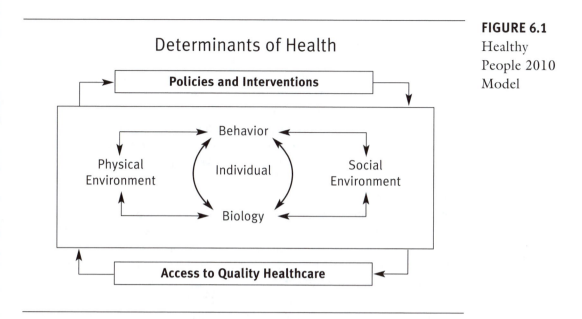

FIGURE 6.1

Healthy
People 2010
Model

Source: U.S. Department of Health and Human Services. 2000. *Healthy People 2010: Understanding and Improving Health, 2nd edition.* [Online document; retrieved 12/12/05.] www.healthypeople.gov /Document/tableofcontents.htm#under.

including to "purchase health care; provide health care; ensure access to quality care for vulnerable populations; regulate health care markets; support acquisition of new knowledge; develop and evaluate health technologies and practices; monitor health care quality; inform health care decision makers; develop the health care workforce; and, convene stakeholder from across the health care system" (Tang, Eisenberg, and Meyer 2004, 47). Within each of these functions are numerous strategies designed to accomplish the intended purpose. For instance, a myriad of quality oversight organizations operate from national, state, and local levels to assess and monitor the quality of healthcare organizations, services, and professionals. Figure 6.2 summarizes these organizations and their respective roles.

Federal Healthcare-Quality Reporting Initiatives

In 1987, the Health Care Financing Agency (HCFA), now known as the Centers for Medicare and Medicaid Services or CMS, produced its first annual report of "observed hospital-specific mortality rates for Medicare acute care hospitals" (Cleves and Golden 1996, 40). The mortality data represented early efforts of HCFA's Effectiveness Initiative, the goal of which was to produce "better information to guide the decisions of physicians, patients and the agency, thus improving outcomes and the quality of care" (Roper et al. 1988, 1198). The initiative consisted of the following components:

FIGURE 6.2
Quality
Oversight in
Healthcare

Roles of Quality Oversight Organizations
Quality Oversight Organizations are organizations that assess the quality of
health care delivered by health plans, facilities, and integrated delivery systems, as well as individual practitioners. These organizations include both private gateway.html organizations as well as Federal, State, and local government agencies. Although they vary widely in the scope of their reviews as well
as the types of action they can take, they represent a concentration of expertise and knowledge that can be used to improve health care. They include:

State Licensing Bodies
States, typically through their health departments, have long regulated health
care delivery through the licensure of health care institutions such as hospitals,
long-term care facilities, and home health agencies, as well as individual health
care practitioners such as physicians and nurses. States also license, through
their insurance and health departments, financial "risk-bearing entities,"
including both indemnity insurance products and those managed care products
that perform the dual function of bearing risk (like an insurer) and arranging for
or delivering health care services (like health care–providing entities).

Private Sector Accrediting Bodies
Accrediting bodies set standards for health care organizations and assess
compliance with those standards. They also focus on the operation and effec-
tiveness of internal quality improvement systems. In some areas, State and
Federal governments rely on or recognize private accreditation for purposes of
ensuring compliance with licensure or regulatory requirements. Existing
accreditation efforts include:
- For managed care plans: The National Committee for Quality Assurance
  (NCQA), the Joint Commission on Accreditation of Health Care
  Organizations (JCAHO), and the American Accreditation Health Care
  Commission/Utilization Review Accreditation Commission (AAHCC/URAC);
- For hospitals: JCAHO, the American Osteopathic Association (for osteo-
  pathic hospitals), and the Rehabilitation Accreditation Commission (for
  rehabilitation hospitals);
- Behavioral health organizations: JCAHO (for institutions and behavioral health
  organizations) and NCQA (for managed behavioral health organizations);
- Long-term care facilities: JCAHO;
- Home care organizations: JCAHO and the Community Health Accreditation
  Program of the National League of Nursing;
- Ambulatory care organizations: JCAHO and the Accreditation Association
  for Ambulatory Health Care (AAAHC);
- Clinical laboratories: JCAHO and the College of American Pathologists;
- Physicians: The American Medical Association recently launched a volun-
  tary accreditation program (the American Medical Accreditation Program)
  to measure and evaluate individual physicians against national standards.
  In addition, medical specialty certifying boards already have established
  methods to evaluate cognitive knowledge in board certification and recerti-

continued

FIGURE 6.2
(Continued)

fication. Some of these organizations also have begun approaches to proficiency testing for specific clinical skills and performance measures.

Medicare, Medicaid Compliance
In order for a health care entity to receive Medicare or Medicaid reimbursement, the entity must meet certain federally specified "Conditions of Participation" (COPs) or other standards. The U.S. Health Care Financing Administration (HCFA)* promulgates COPs for hospitals, home health agencies, nursing facilities, hospices, ambulatory surgical centers, renal dialysis centers, rural health clinics, outpatient physical and occupation therapy, and rehabilitation facilities. HCFA also establishes standards for the participation of managed care organizations contracting under the Medicare program.

Department of Labor
Oversight of certain aspects of employer-provided health plans is performed by the U.S. Department of Labor. The Employee Retirement Income Security Act of 1974 sets minimum Federal standards for group health plans maintained by private sector employers, unions, or jointly by employers and unions. The Department oversees plan compliance with the following legal requirements of plan administration: reporting and disclosure of plan features and operations, fiduciary obligations for management of the plan and its assets, handling benefit claims, continuation coverage for workers who lose group health coverage, limitations on exclusions for pre-existing conditions, prohibitions on discrimination based on health status, renewability of group health coverage for employers, minimum hospital stays for childbirth, and parity of limits on mental health benefits.

Individual Certification and Credentialing Organizations
The American Board of Medical Specialties (an umbrella for 24 specialty boards) and the American Osteopathic Association have certification programs that designate certain medical providers as having completed specific training in a specialty and having passed examinations testing knowledge of that specialty. The Accreditation Council for Graduate Medical Education, sponsored by the American Medical Association and four other organizations, accredits nearly 7,700 residency programs in 1,600 medical institutions across the country. For nursing, the American Board of Nursing Specialties sets standards for the certification of nursing specialties. The largest numbers of nurses, both in generalist and specialist practice, are certified by the American Nurses Credentialling Center, based on practice standards established by the American Nurses Association.

*Note: since the publication of this report, the Health Care Financing Administration has been renamed the Centers for Medicare and Medicaid Services.

Source: President's Advisory Committee on Consumer Protection and Quality in the Health Care Industry. 1998. "Quality First: Better Health Care for All Americans." [Online information; retrieved 8/6/05.] www.hcqualitycommission.gov/final/.

> First…using data from the Medicare systems of claims processing
> and peer review to monitor trends and assess the effectiveness of
> specific interventions…. Second, plans for a data resource center
> are being developed and files of Medicare data are being made
> available for appropriate research by private persons and organiza-
> tions…. Third, clinical research is being funded, both intramurally
> and extramurally, that will examine the appropriateness and effec-
> tiveness of various procedures…. Finally, the methods of conduct-
> ing research on effectiveness are being improved and the data
> bases expanded (Roper et al. 1988, 1198).

The mortality data reports were discontinued in 1994 and the focus
turned to high-volume, high-cost clinical conditions. Between 1997 and
1999, HCFA collected quality process measures on acute myocardial
infarction (AMI), breast cancer, diabetes mellitus, congestive heart failure (CHF), pneumonia, and stroke. Noteworthy about the study was that
unlike the mortality data derived from administrative claims data, these
data were abstracted directly from the Medicare patients' clinical records.
The aim was not only to compare effectiveness of care on a national level
but also to establish a reliable methodology for collecting quality process
measures for which there was "strong scientific evidence and professional
consensus either directly improves outcomes or is a necessary step in a
chain of care that does so" (Jencks et al. 2000, 1670). Study results
showed how each state performed in the 24 clinical process measures
(Jencks et al. 2000).

In 2003, a follow-up study was published, which showed performance in 22 of 24 of the original measures during 2000 through 2001 (Jencks,
Huff, and Cuerdon 2003). By 2004, CMS had established the voluntary
reporting initiative where eligible hospitals could voluntarily report their
performance on quality indicators in the three conditions of AMI, CHF,
and community-acquired pneumonia. By 2005, hospitals providing care
for Medicare patients and receiving reimbursement from CMS (excluding
critical access hospitals) were required to submit their performance data
on the designated measures to CMS. In 2005, hospital-specific results were
posted on the U.S. Department of Health and Human Services website
called "Hospital Compare" for public access and review.

Concurrent with the CMS Hospital Quality Initiative were efforts
to define, collect, and publish quality indicators for nursing homes and
home health agencies. At the time of this writing, plans are under way to
add new measures to the clinical data set in prevention of surgical wound
infection, to introduce a satisfaction survey—the Hospital Consumer
Assessment of Healthcare Providers and Systems, and to expand quality
reporting to the ambulatory care setting. The unit of analysis, which has
already evolved from the state level to the hospital level, will be continually refined to the provider level.

JCAHO Initiatives

Federal efforts to make clinical performance data available to the public were complemented by private efforts through JCAHO. In 2002, JCAHO "implemented evidence-based standardized measures of performance in over 3000 accredited hospitals. The measures were designed to track hospitals' performance over time and encourage improvement through quarterly feedback in the form of comparative reports to all participating hospitals" (Williams et al. 2005, 256).

Performance measures are one component of JCAHO's redesigned approach to accreditation. Just as in the scenario in Chapter 1, JCAHO realized the pitfalls of the traditional accreditation process and has aggressively introduced changes that require health services organizations to move along the quality continuum if they are to fulfill accreditation requirements. Started in 1999 and officially launched in 2004, JCAHO's Shared Visions–New Pathways accreditation process is described as "a paradigm shift from a process focused on survey preparation to one of continuous systematic and operational improvement by focusing to a greater extent on the provision of safe, high quality care, treatment and services" (Joint Commission and Joint Commission Resources 2004, 1).

The redesigned approach to accreditation includes revised and streamlined accreditation standards, use of organizational data to tailor the accreditation process to the organization's specific needs and patient population, a focus on continuous compliance by combining on-site surveys with online compliance documentation, enhanced electronic communication between JCAHO and health services organizations, and use of the tracer methodology for on-site surveys (Joint Commission Resources 2003).

In the past, surveyors focused on documents as the source of information to determine an organization's compliance with JCAHO standards. These documents included policies, procedures, administrative records, and patients' clinical charts. The redesigned process focuses on direct observation and discussions with care providers, other frontline employees, and patients as well as real-time document review as the primary sources of information.

JCAHO has also changed to an on-site survey process called the *tracer methodology*, which provides the opportunity to examine both the depth and breadth of an organization's quality and safety efforts. For example, infection control, medication management, data use, and environment of care are such key areas influencing patient quality and safety that JCAHO has designated them as priority areas for in-depth evaluation within and across departments in the organization. In a *system tracer*, the surveyor examines the multiple processes, systems, and structures that make up these priority areas. For example, a system tracer for medication management would include processes for how an organization selects, stores, orders,

FIGURE 6.3

System and
Individual
Tracers

System Tracer
The surveyor "traces" the elements of the system.

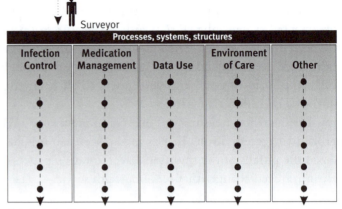

Note: Dashed vertical arrows reflect standards evaluation opportunities related to exploration of the design of a system and the dots represent any given elements of a system.

Individual Tracer
The surveyor "traces" the course of care provided to the recipient.

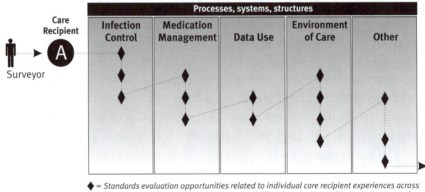

◆ = Standards evaluation opportunities related to individual care recipient experiences across multiple functions (for example, dispensing and administration in medication management).

Source: © Joint Commission Resources: *Tracer Methodology: Tips and Strategies for Continuous Systems Improvement.* Oakbrook Terrace, IL: Joint Commission on Accreditation of Healthcare Organizations, 2004, pp. 5–6. Reprinted with permission.

dispenses, and administers medications as well as how the providers evaluate effectiveness of drug therapy and identify, track, and prevent adverse drug events. The system tracer methodology takes into account the "set of components that work together toward a common goal…and how well the organization's systems function. This approach addresses the interrelationships of the many elements that go into delivering safe, high-quality care and translates standards compliance issues into potential organizational vulnerabilities" (Cockshut-Miller 2004, 14). Figure 6.3 shows a schematic of the system tracer approach.

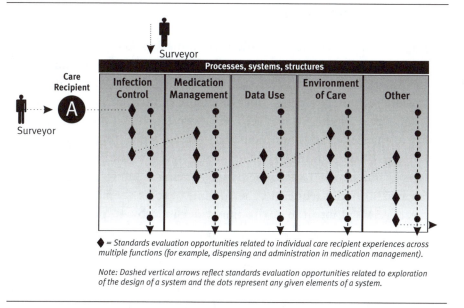

FIGURE 6.4

Combined
System and
Individual
Tracers

◆ = *Standards evaluation opportunities related to individual care recipient experiences across multiple functions (for example, dispensing and administration in medication management).*

Note: Dashed vertical arrows reflect standards evaluation opportunities related to exploration of the design of a system and the dots represent any given elements of a system.

Source: © Joint Commission Resources: *Tracer Methodology: Tips and Strategies for Continuous Systems Improvement.* Oakbrook Terrace, IL: Joint Commission on Accreditation of Healthcare Organizations, 2004, pp. 5–6. Reprinted with permission.

While a system tracer follows one of the priority areas throughout the organization, an individual tracer follows a patient's experience within the organization. Surveyors evaluate how the actual delivery of care is executed in a manner that complies with standards within the context of the patient's progression through the episode of care. Based on the data collected about the organization before the survey, a patient condition is selected. When the surveyors arrive on site, an actual patient is chosen from the current patient census. Questions are posed to staff currently caring for this patient and to staff in all of the other departments who have interacted or may interact with this patient during her current stay or visit. "Just as individual's care encompass[es] several standards at one time, surveyors focus on a number of related processes of care rather than just one process...for example, re-assessment, nutrition, medical equipment risks, and caregiver competencies might all be considered when tracing the care of a resident in a long term care facility.... [U]nder the new accreditation process, it is not as important for staff to know what the...standard is, but rather to know how they provide safe, high-quality care, treatment and services to individuals" (Joint Commission Resources 2004, 10). Figure 6.3 shows a schematic of an individual tracer.

Figure 6.4 illustrates the complementary nature of these two types of tracers used in the survey process and how, when used together, they provide a comprehensive picture of the organization's systems approach to quality and safety.

A Systems Approach

During the time since the initial Medicare mortality data reports, CMS has systematically developed and implemented the expectations, requirements, methodology, and infrastructure to collect, publish, and disseminate clinical-quality performance data. Public disclosure or "transparency" has proven to be an effective strategy to reduce risk for consumers and promote accountability of businesses in other industries. For example, "in 1986 Congress passed a new law requiring manufacturers to reveal to the public their toxic releases in standardized form, chemical by chemical and factory by factory" (Graham 2002). Subsequently, the amount of toxic chemicals that manufacturers released into the environment declined by 46 percent between the years 1988 and 1999. Although this example is relatively recent, public disclosure has a long history in the United States. The Securities and Exchange Acts passed in the 1930s required publicly traded companies to publish earnings data. These two examples illustrate the power of information as a "regulatory mechanism" (Graham 2002).

While arguably, the healthcare industry is unique compared to securities and environmental pollution, the common theme is the potential of information to reduce risk to consumers, particularly in a market economy. When one considers the statistics about the current state of quality in the U.S. healthcare system, provided in Figure 1.1 as "risks" to patients, providers, organizations, payers, and employers, one begins to gain an appreciation for the growing interest and activity directed toward reducing risk through public disclosure of health quality data.

In the early description of the HCFA Effectiveness Initiative, Roper, the director of HCFA at the time, explains why this type of effort must be undertaken by the federal agency. He states that "information about the effectiveness of particular services provides a public good.... [H]owever, because the benefit of better information accrues to the public at large, not just to those collecting it, the market system may not ensure adequate investment in the necessary research and data collection" (Roper et al. 1988, 1197).

The federal healthcare-quality reporting initiatives illustrate an understanding of a systems approach to improving health outcomes by targeting the effect of policy requirements on individual, organizational behavior, and community behavior; the relationship of performance data transparency and accountability; and the role of performance measurement in better understanding and improving system behavior.

The new accreditation approach by JCAHO, in particular the tracer methodology, illustrates a systems approach by focusing on the interrelatedness of the numerous patient care processes and how accreditation standards may cut across numerous departments, processes, and areas within health services organizations. A focus on continuous—rather than periodic—compliance encourages organizations to progress along the quality continuum described in Chapter 1.

Both JCAHO and CMS recognize the importance of a unified and aligned approach at the public-policy and private-policy levels and are collaborating to align measures and methodologies with common disease categories. Through its conditions for participation and conditions for coverage, CMS (2005) "also ensures that the standards of accrediting organizations recognized by CMS (through a process called 'deeming') meet or exceed Medicare standards." As CMS continues to pursue reimbursement schemes based on performance measures, the relationship between financial incentives and quality is also being targeted to drive overall health system improvement.

Conclusion

A brief introduction is provided in this chapter about the role of public and private policies in fueling the imperative for improving quality in health services. Because of the dynamic and rapidly changing nature of this topic, readers are encouraged to review the accompanying Internet resources as a means to keep current on changes, new initiatives, and plans for the future. The exercise at the end of the chapter is designed to familiarize readers with the CMS website.

Chapter 7 addresses another aspect of the systems approach: the concept of systemic structure in organizations.

Companion Readings

Jha, A. K., Z. Li, E. J. Orav, and A. M. Epstein. 2005. "Care in U.S. Hospitals—The Hospital Quality Alliance Program." *New England Journal of Medicine* 353 (3): 265–74.

Roper, W. L., W. Winkenwerder, G. M. Hackbarth, and H. Krakauer. 1988. "Effectiveness in Health Care: An Initiative to Evaluate and Improve Medical Practice." *New England Journal of Medicine* 319: 1197–202.

Williams, S. C., S. P. Schmaltz, D. J. Morton, R. G. Koss, and J. M. Loeb. 2005. "Quality of Care in U.S. Hospitals, as Reflected by Standardized Measures, 2002–2004." *New England Journal of Medicine* 353 (3): 255–64.

Web Resources

Centers for Medicare and Medicaid Services

Quality Initiatives: www.cms.hhs.gov/quality/
Hospital Quality Initiative: www.cms.hhs.gov/quality/hospital/
Hospital Compare: www.hospitalcompare.hhs.gov/

Nursing Home Quality Initiative (with link to Nursing Home Compare):
www.cms.hhs.gov/quality/nhqi/

Home Health Quality Initiative (with link to Home Health Compare):
www.cms.hhs.gov/quality/hhqi/

Physician Focused Quality Initiative (ambulatory care):
www.cms.hhs.gov/quality/pfqi.asp

Joint Commission on Accreditation of Healthcare Organizations

Shared Visions–New Pathways Resources:
www.jointcommission.org/AccreditationPrograms/SVNP/

Quality Check (organization-specific accreditation information and performance data): ww.qualitycheck.org/

Additional Resources

Agency for Healthcare Research and Quality (quality and patient safety):
www.ahrq.gov/qual/

Agency for Healthcare Research and Quality (quality tools):
www.qualitytools.ahrq.gov/

Archived Reports

Quality Interagency Coordination Task Force ("Doing What Counts for Patient Safety: Federal Actions to Reduce Medical Errors and Their Impact"):
www.quic.gov/report/toc.htm

References

Cleves, M. A., and W. E. Golden. 1996. "Assessment of HCFA's 1992 Medicare Hospital Information Report of Mortality Following Admission for Hip Arthroplasty." *Health Services Research* 31 (1): 39–48.

Centers for Medicare and Medicaid Services (CMS). 2005. "Conditions for Participation/Conditions for Coverage." [Online information; retrieved 12/12/05.] www.cms.hhs.gov/cop/default.asp.

Cockshut-Miller, L. (ed.). 2004. *Tracer Methodology: Tips and Strategies for Continuous Systems Improvement.* Oakbrook Terrace, IL: Joint Commission Resources.

Graham, M. 2002. "Is Sunshine the Best Disinfectant? The Promise and Problems of Environmental Disclosure." [Online information; retrieved 5/7/06.] www.brookings.edu/press/review/spring2002/graham.htm.

Jencks, S. F., T. Cuerdon, D. R. Burwen, B. Fleming, P. M. Houck, A. E. Kussmaul, D. S. Nilasena, D. L. Ordin, and D. R. Arday. 2000. "Quality of Medical Care Delivered to Medicare Beneficiaries: A Profile at State and National Levels." *JAMA* 284 (13): 1670–76.

Jencks, S. F., E. D. Huff, and T. Cuerdon. 2003. "Change in the Quality of Care Delivered to Medicare Beneficiaries, 1998–1999 to 2000–2001." *JAMA* 289 (3): 305–12.

Joint Commission Resources. 2003. "Shared Visions–New Pathways: An Innovative Approach to Patient Safety and Quality Improvement." Video. Oakbrook Terrace, IL: Joint Commission on Accreditation of Healthcare Organizations.

Joint Commission and Joint Commission Resources. 2004. "Special Report: JCAHO Shared Visions–New Pathways." *Joint Commission Perspectives, The Official Joint Commission Newsletter* 24 (1): 1–27.

Longest, B. B. 2002. *Health Policy in the United States, 3rd edition.* Chicago: Health Administration Press.

President's Advisory Committee on Consumer Protection and Quality in the Health Care Industry. 1998. "Quality First: Better Health Care for All Americans." [Online information; retrieved 8/6/05.] www.hcqualitycommission.gov/final/.

Roper, W. L., W. Winkenwerder, G. M. Hackbarth, and H. Krakauer. 1988. "Effectiveness in Health Care: An Initiative to Evaluate and Improve Medical Practice." *New England Journal of Medicine* 319 (18): 1197–202.

Tang, N., J. M. Eisenberg, and G. S. Meyer. 2004. "The Roles of Government in Improving Health Care Quality and Safety." *Joint Commission Journal on Quality and Safety* 30 (4): 47–55.

U.S. Department of Health and Human Services. 2000. *Healthy People 2010: Understanding and Improving Health, 2nd edition.* [Online publication; retrieved 12/12/05.] www.healthypeople.gov/Document /tableofcontents.htm#under.

Williams, S. C., S. P. Schmaltz, D. J. Morton, R. G. Koss, and J. M. Loeb. 2005. "Quality of Care in U.S. Hospitals, as Reflected by Standardized Measures, 2002–2004." *New England Journal of Medicine* 353 (3): 255–64.

Exercise

Objective: To become familiar with the CMS quality initiatives.

Instructions

1. Based on your work setting and/or area of interest, select and explore one of CMS quality initiatives (e.g., hospitals, home health, nursing home) at www.cms.hhs.gov/quality.
2. Answer the following questions in reference to the selected resource:
   a. In two to three paragraphs, describe the contents of this resource and its relationship to healthcare quality.
   b. Describe how the information contained on this site may be used in your current or previous organizational setting.
   c. Choose, analyze, and interpret one data set contained in this resource. Explain what these data mean in the context of healthcare quality.

SYSTEMIC STRUCTURE

Objectives

- To introduce the metaphor of an iceberg to help demonstrate the concept of systemic structure in organizations
- To discuss practical lessons for healthcare managers resulting from understanding the concept of systemic structure
- To introduce strategies to help managers identify and understand systemic structures
- To practice identifying different mental models or assumptions in healthcare and understanding how they influence behavior

On Thursday, Nurse Smith volunteers to work a double shift in the ICU. The next day, he misses his regularly scheduled shift when he calls in sick. The following month, Nurse Jones, who works in the same ICU, volunteers to work a double shift. Two days later, she misses her regularly scheduled shift when she calls in sick. When the ICU manager mentions this "coincidence" to his colleagues, they also describe similar situations on their respective units. As the ICU manager gathers more information about employee staffing practices, he realizes that, although the policies help staffing in the short term, the same policies inadvertently contribute to increased sick calls and more overtime in the long run.

The manager was discovering that well-intended efforts, such as the carefully written policies and procedures for his department, may not yield expected results. Likewise, well-intended change or improvement interventions often yield disappointing results. This chapter begins to explore how a systems perspective can help managers improve the quality of organizational interventions.

A Systems Metaphor for Organizations

Metaphors can be a valuable tool because they provide a concrete picture of a theoretical concept (Armenakis and Bedian 1992; Clearly and Packard 1992); after the concept has been translated into a tangible form, it becomes easier to understand and remember. Thinking of an organization as an iceberg is one metaphor that illustrates the subtle but powerful systems

FIGURE 7.1

The Iceberg
Metaphor

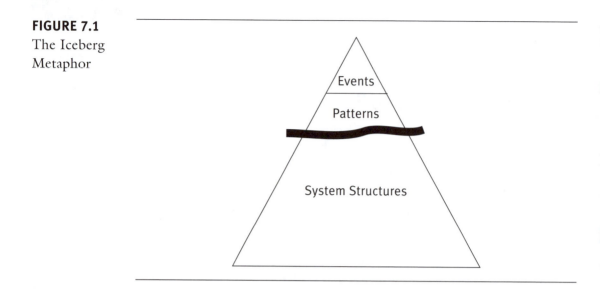

Source: Reprinted with permission from Innovations Associates, Inc. 1995. "Systems Thinking: A Language for Learning and Action." Participant manual, version 95.4.1. Waltham, Massachusetts.

principles at work in organizations (Innovation Associates, Inc. 1995). Like an iceberg, where nine-tenths of the iceberg's mass is underwater (GLACIER 2003), the essence of an organization's makeup is not visible to most observers. Those forces that cause an organization to function the way it does and the people in the organization to behave the way they do may not be readily observable. Yet just as the part of the iceberg that is beneath the water's surface is dangerous to passing ships, what is below the organizational "waterline" can sink well-intended change and improvement efforts.

The triangular shape in Figure 7.1 represents the iceberg, and the wavy, thick line represents the waterline. The tip of the iceberg (the top layer of the triangle) represents the events that occur daily in the organization. The middle layer of the iceberg represents a deeper understanding of the organization as a system by linking events into patterns of behavior. The bottom level of the iceberg, which is underwater, represents the deepest understanding of the behavior of the organization as a system. This level represents relationships among variables in the system that cause the events and patterns to occur.

In the staffing example at the beginning of this chapter, the nurse managers observed the nurses working double shifts and calling in sick as independent events on each of their units. However, while comparing notes, they identified a pattern of behavior across three different patient care units. Although the act of identifying patterns is still above the organizational waterline, it is the first step toward systems thinking. The manager began to go below the waterline when he identified relationships between the observations and patterns. By telling a "story" of his discoveries, the relationships and underlying causes of the problems began to emerge. This was the story:

> The hospital policies were supposed to promote adequate staffing and discourage sick calls; however, the day shifts were often over-staffed and the evening and nights shifts were understaffed.
>
> Nurses were paid overtime and often an additional "premium" for working a double shift. When nurses volunteered for a double shift, they were positively perceived as "helpful" and "team players." The nurse helped out with a shift that was short-staffed and did not, in turn, cause a shift to be short-staffed by calling in sick.
>
> By working a double shift and calling in sick later in the week, the nurses were able to work the same amount of hours but get paid for four more hours than if they had worked their regularly sched-uled shifts.

The manager was beginning to see the relationships among the key variables in the system: scheduling policies, individual employee incentives, compensation and rewards, sick-call policy, individual unit operations, and float pool operations. Although individually the policies and operations seemed reasonable, their interactions with each other contributed to the underlying systemic structure: the relationship between the perceived ben-efit to nurses (i.e., helping out peers and patients, earning the same money while working fewer hours, or earning more money while working the same hours) and the frequency of the behavior of volunteering for a double shift and calling in sick later in the week. These two variables were related in a way that reinforced the behavior—that is, as the number of nurses who perceived this benefit increased, the number of times the behavior occurred increased. Note that the nurses had no malicious intent in this case; they were simply following the policies as they were crafted. As this reinforcing relationship occurred across several nursing departments, however, the unintended result to the hospital was an overall increase in salary expense.

Only when the manager understood each of the policies within the context of how they made up the whole were he and other managers able to redesign the system to achieve the intended result of staffing the hospital in a dependable and cost-effective manner. Some of the changes this organiza-tion made to break the reinforcing cycle included reviewing the distribution of nurses during the day, evening, and night shifts to better balance staffing across the 24-hour period; improving coordination between the nursing unit schedules and the float pool's schedules; and changing the overtime criteria (consistent with legal labor requirements) from hours worked in excess of eight hours per day to hours worked in excess of 40 hours per week.

Lessons for Healthcare Managers

When using the iceberg metaphor to describe an organization, events and patterns may be thought of as occurring above the waterline. The term "systemic structure" refers to what is found below the waterline. The systemic structure involves the interrelationships among key variables within the system and the influence of these interrelationships on the system's behavior over time (Senge 1990). Note that systemic structure refers to interrelationships among variables in the system and not to interpersonal relationships among people. Systemic structure should also be differentiated from organizational structure, which refers to how responsibility and authority are distributed throughout an organization (Shortell and Kaluzny 2000).

Valuable insights about organizations may be gained by understanding the concept of systemic structure. This section offers four lessons for healthcare managers that have resulted from these insights:

1.   Systemic structure influences behavior.
2.   Systemic structure is invisible.
3.   Information is essential to identifying systemic structure.
4.   Successful change requires going below the waterline.

Lesson 1: Systemic Structure Influences Behavior

Consider the following story from an anonymous author:

> A college student spent an entire summer going to the football field every day wearing a black-and-white striped shirt, walking up and down the field for ten or fifteen minutes, throwing bird seed all over the field, blowing a whistle, and then walking off the field. At the end of the summer, it came time for the first home football game. The referee walked onto the field and blew the whistle. The game had to be delayed for a half hour to wait for the birds to get off the field.

Everyone laughs at this story. However, if one were sitting in the stadium stands without a clue about the events of the summer, one would probably be annoyed and blame those darn birds. The birds were not right or wrong. They were doing exactly what they were supposed to be doing based on the underlying systemic structures: the relationships between feeding time and the football field, the striped shirt and the bird seed, the whistle and their hunger. Similar situations occur with providers and employees in health services organizations. The thought of a healthcare professional coming to work to intentionally do a poor job seems absurd. However, the desire to blame is often an initial management response to a negative situation or a medical error.

"Every organization is perfectly designed to get the results that it gets. To get different result you need to improve the design of the organization"

(Hanna 1988, 36). This expression has become common in quality improvement presentations and articles. However, what is not commonly heard or read is that design needs to be improved not only above the waterline but also below the waterline. The phrase "every organization is perfectly designed to get the results that it gets" is usually applied within the context of events (i.e., the top level of the iceberg). When improvements are designed from the event level, managers and providers will typically ask, "What do we need to do differently? What actions (e.g., implementing clinical guidelines, streamlining office scheduling systems, installing new computers) will bring us closer to our vision of quality healthcare?"

An understanding of the iceberg metaphor, however, shows that questions must be asked from all levels of the iceberg, from observing events to determining patterns in the events to identifying underlying structures that cause the patterns and events to occur. This changing view also alters the questions the managers and providers must ask. Rather than focusing only on "What can we do differently?" managers must also ask, "How can we best understand why we are getting the results we are getting?" The manager will then begin to look for patterns in recurrent events, try to understand how past events may be contributing to current behavior, and begin to uncover the key relationships among variables that are influencing current behavior of the system. Only when this has been done can the manager target interventions that alter these relationships and that in turn lead to sustainable improvements in the actions intended to deliver better organizational and patient results.

The iceberg metaphor adds insight to issues on an industry level as well as on the organizational level. For example, in the 1990s changing work conditions from hospital restructuring and downsizing led nurses in Victoria, Australia, to change from

> full-time to part-time work because they couldn't cope with the strain of working full-time…because hospitals were having trouble getting nurses to work for them, temporary agencies stepped in to fill the gap. But this simply exacerbated the shortage…. Agencies were paying their nurses three times the amount of money permanent staff were getting…so more and more nurses left permanent work in the hospital and went and worked agency…. [I]nstead of rewarding permanent nurses to fill in schedule deficits, nurse managers were going to agency nurses…. [T]he permanent staff saw that the agency nurse was getting flexibility, shifts they wanted to work, and also more pay. So they left permanent work for agency work…. [C]osts of agency nurses rose from $30 million to $55 million a year (Gordon 2005, 346).

Similar relationships among healthcare restructuring, work conditions, temporary agencies, and management philosophies have explained nationwide nurse shortages in the United States, Canada, and the United Kingdom (Gordon 2005).

Lesson 2: Systemic Structure Is Invisible

Systemic structure is usually invisible unless a conscious effort is made to find it. As with an iceberg, just because managers do not see what is below the organizational waterline does not mean that systemic structure is not present in the organization. For example, a newly hired manager at an academic medical center was assigned to facilitate an improvement project on one patient care unit. If the project proved successful on this unit, the intent was to expand the intervention organizationwide. Despite positive results—as measured by improved cycle times, increased patient satisfaction, and increased staff satisfaction—the project was not implemented beyond the original pilot site. When the manager began to explore possible reasons that the project was not replicated on the other units, she discovered that over the years numerous project teams had designed and implemented successful pilot projects aimed at improving specific problems. However, very few of these projects had actually been integrated into the ongoing activities of the organization (i.e., institutionalized).

Upon further investigation, she uncovered the following systemic structures operating in this organization. First, all improvements in the organization were called "pilots." The expectation was that a trial would be conducted for a specified period, that results would be presented to the administrative team, and that the administrative team would then authorize the project to continue or not. The problem was that this process occurred independently from the budgeting process. When the "special pools" of dollars to fund a pilot were gone, no mechanisms were in place to reallocate funds either within or among departments to support a successful improvement or innovation.

The pilot label also brought with it other short-term perceptions related to support, staffing, and budgets. Because of these invisible, but real, relationships among the variables required to support change, this academic medical center demonstrated a constant stream of successful improvement pilot efforts yet wondered why sustained improvement in the overall organizational performance never occurred.

Lesson 3: Information Is Essential to Identifying Systemic Structure

The dictionary defines a pattern as "a consistent, characteristic form, style, or method; composite of traits or features characteristic of an individual or a group." This definition implies that identifying or recognizing a pattern requires more than one observation. In the nurse staffing example, the discussion among the nurse managers about issues on their respective units provided an opportunity to observe behavior of many nurses across multiple units. Only when these observations were combined did the organizational pattern become evident.

The need for multiple observations or data points has implications for how managers determine organizational structure, interact and communicate, and present performance data. The traditional vertical organizational structure, which compartmentalizes groups within rigid reporting lines, reduces the opportunity to interact across departments and disciplines and reduces the opportunity to identify organizational patterns. Communication methods based on "telling" rather than "sharing" information also reduce the opportunity to identify organizational patterns by reducing two-way communication and the "fresh eyes" often needed to interpret and link events. Data reported by single time periods only (e.g., monthly departmental financial reports) reduce managers' ability to identify patterns over time in their own departments; on the other hand, aggregated, organizational data reduce managers' opportunity to identify patterns across smaller units of analysis within the organization.

Strategies that can promote pattern identification and prompt investigation into underlying structures include

- organizational structures and/or cultures that encourage interaction among levels and units,
- open and free flow of information, and
- performance data displayed on run charts or control charts to make data trends over time more visible. (Chapter 9 further explores the role of measurement in pattern identification.)

Lesson 4: Successful Change Requires Going Below the Waterline

To implement successful and lasting change efforts, managers must go below the organizational waterline. An understanding of the iceberg metaphor explains why the potential of many change or improvement efforts is not fully realized. If changes are targeted at the event or pattern levels (i.e., what we do) rather than at the systemic structure level (i.e., what causes the system to behave the way it does), the impact will only be temporary. Because structure influences behavior, the only way to truly change behavior within the system is to identify, target, and change the underlying structures.

There is no shortage of ideas on how to improve organizational systems; however, a common challenge for managers and care providers alike is how to actually implement these ideas. Organizational culture may be thought of as an underlying systemic structure. The influence of hospital culture on the ability to convert CQI concepts into effective implementation has been described in the healthcare research literature (Shortell et al. 1995). Another example may be seen in the area of clinical practice guidelines. Although providers generally support evidence-based practice, translating evidence into practice has historically been difficult to achieve

(Cabana et al. 1999; Solberg 2002). In recent years, health services researchers have studied the role of systemic structures, such as leadership, context, and incentives, in guideline implementation (McCormack et al. 2002; Solberg 2000a, 2000b). The CMS quality initiatives described in the previous chapter target underlying structures, such as financial incentives, recognition, and status.

Going Below the Waterline

The captain of a ship sailing in the North Atlantic uses radar, a sonar, and a bow watch (a sailor posted at the front of the ship to look out for danger) to alert him to underwater ice. Likewise, managers may also use strategies that alert them to underlying systemic structures. Following are three strategies managers may use:
1. Understanding history
2. Being aware of mental models
3. Integrating double-loop learning into their management philosophy and approach

Understanding History

History is a powerful underlying structure. A healthcare manager's current work may be influenced by her department's history, the hospital's history, a professional group's history, the community's history, or the industry's history. For example, the sudden death of a well-respected department manager had a long-lasting impact on the department staff. The new incumbent manager was faced not only with getting settled in a new role and new department but also with addressing the staff's grief. For new employees, the lack of shared history with the deceased manager was a source of polarization between the "before" and "after" staff and interfered with the entire staff's ability to achieve a high level of teamwork.

A nurse at a rehabilitation center that had recently been purchased by a "for-profit" organization carefully explained the organization's history to a patient's family. The previous owners and managers of the center were proud of their heritage of religious service and quality. The family inquired if their family member would still get what she needed at this for-profit facility, and the nurse informed the family that the staff still identified with the center's historic values.

In the book *The Social Transformation of American Medicine*, Paul Starr (1982) describes the evolution of the U.S. medical profession and physicians' roles from the eighteenth century through the twentieth century. Although one may agree or disagree with Starr's conclusions, this book explains how the history of physicians, hospitals, and insurance companies shaped the healthcare industry of today, and as such the book provides a level of understanding of the current state of our healthcare system. Understanding the circumstances surrounding the Flexner report, which was published in 1910 and describes the state of medical education at the time, can provide insights into why medical schools are structured the way they are and into the role of academic medical centers in U.S. healthcare. Understanding the numerous occasions that national health insurance has been on the political agenda (1917, the 1930s, and the 1940s) as well as the American Medical Association's role in those debates can provide insight into physicians' responses to contemporary issues surrounding healthcare reform (Starr 1982).

The simplest strategies that managers may use to understand history are to ask, listen, and read. In addition, approaches to large-group "visioning" meetings have incorporated structured discussions about history (Weisbord 1987). Managers, especially those assuming a new role, may gain valuable insights by facilitating similar discussions with staff in their own departments. The following guidelines may help:

- Ask the group to identify significant events during defined periods. Events within the department, organization, community, clinical specialty or profession, or industry may be identified.
- List the events by periods of time (e.g., in five- or ten-year increments, depending on the group).
- Look for patterns in the listed events.

For example, one group of nurses in the postpartum area identified this event in their history discussion: At 5:00 every morning, the charge nurse would announce over the unit's intercom system, "Patients who have not had a bowel movement yet, please put on your nurse call light." The group burst into laughter, and one nurse observed, "Glad those 'good old days' are gone!" This simple observation helped the group to let go of its resistance to a proposed change on the unit as it realized that it had experienced numerous changes over the years, most of which had direct benefit to the patients.

A manager in a laboratory was intrigued about the type of events identified during the history discussion with staff. Most of the identified events focused on current events from the news, and few events focused on laboratory technology or the department, as he had anticipated. The manager realized that because the demographic composition of his department had been changing over the years (the technologists were 40 years old or older, the technical assistants and phlebotomists were 30 years old or younger), the two distinct demographics had little in common to talk about but current events. This realization not only helped to explain why previous team-building sessions had only been moderately successful but also prompted the manager to establish common ground for his employees through a shared vision for the department. This manager also became more attentive to age diversity, succession planning, and the needs of differing demographic groups, particularly in his approaches to recruitment and hiring (Kelly 1999).

Being Aware of Mental Models

The term "mental model" is often used interchangeably with the terms "paradigm" and "assumption." Although these terms are technically slightly different, they all refer to a deeply ingrained way of thinking that influences how a person sees and understands the world as well as how that person acts. When someone declares an unquestionable status or condition, a mental model is usually being expressed; words like "always" and "never" are clues that mental models are being expressed. Mental models may be so strong that they override the facts at hand. For example, at a quality management workshop, one hospital manager stated her mental model as follows: "Physicians would never spend time at a workshop like this." However, sitting beside her for the duration of the workshop were two pediatricians and a family practitioner!

What this manager did not realize was that her own mental model was interfering with her ability to design appropriate strategies to engage physicians in improvement efforts in her own organization. As a result of her mental model, she found numerous reasons why physicians would not participate and was blinded to strategies to encourage physician participation. To promote learning and improvement in organizations, managers, care providers, and other employees in the organization must "look inward...to reflect critically on their own behavior, identify ways they often inadvertently contribute to the organization's problems, and then change how they act" (Argyris 1991). Without an understanding of our own mental models, we run the risk of unknowingly undermining our own efforts to progress along the quality continuum.

For example, the mental model of "clinical guidelines are used to control physician behavior" encourages organizations to adopt top-down mandates for "cookbook" processes. Alternatively, the mental model of "using evidence-based clinical guidelines to standardize steps of care can actually save physician time on routine interventions so that more time can be spent on the unique needs of the patient" encourages organizations to support and foster clinician involvement in evaluating, selecting, adapting, and implementing clinical guidelines. The mental model of "data are necessary to 'name, blame, and shame'" encourages managers to use data to justify punitive actions. The mental model of "information is power" encourages managers to guard data tightly and to distribute them only on a "need to know" basis. Alternatively, the mental model of "data are the foundation of performance improvement" encourages organizations to put in place information collection, analysis, and dissemination systems that make data easily accessible. Once mental models and their subsequent actions are understood, managers may purposely choose to operate from mental models that help rather than hinder in achieving desired performance results.

Differing mental models may also be a source of conflict within an organization. A manager's view or perspective on organizations themselves

Organizational Characteristic	Rational Model	Political Model
Goals, preferences	Consistent across members	Inconsistent, pluralistic within the organization
Power and control	Centralized	Diffuse, shifting coalitions and interest groups
Decision process	Logical, orderly, sequential	Disorderly, give and take of competing interests
Information	Extensive, systematic, accurate	Ambiguous, selectively available, used as a power resource
Cause-and-effect relationships	Predictable	Uncertain
Decisions	Based on outcome-maximizing choice	Results from bargaining and interplay among interests
Ideology	Efficiency and effectiveness	Struggle, conflict, winners and losers

TABLE 7.1

Comparison of Organizational Models

Source: From *Health Care Management: Organization Design and Behavior,* 4th edition, by S. M. Shortell and A. D. Kaluzny. © 2000. Reprinted with permission of Delmar Learning, a division of Thomson Learning: www.thomsonrights.com. Fax 800 730-2215.

will shape his or her management strategies, actions, and style. Two contrasting views of organizations are the rational model and political model, which are shown in Table 7.1 and are illustrated in the following example.

A manager who viewed organizations through a rational model was extremely frustrated with and ineffective in an organization that operated from a political perspective. From the manager's point of view, the decision-making processes in this politically driven organization served the interest of the players involved but did not result in optimal patient outcomes or cost-effective approaches. On the other hand, the administrative team perceived this manager's emphasis on results as interfering with the delicate political alliances they had worked very hard to establish. The lack of understanding of each other's mental models created ongoing conflict between the manager and the administrative team: The manager thought the team did not care about results, and the team thought the manager was compromising relationships with important stakeholders. Without an awareness of each other's mental models, the conflict between the manager and the administrators continued to grow until the manager finally left the organization.

Had both parties made their mental models explicit—whether through discussion, definition of organizational operating principles, or orientation of new managers to the culture of decision making—their conflict may have been avoided or at least some common understanding may have been established. Instead, the results were conflict, tension, and, eventually, manager turnover.

Because values such as "patient-focused excellence, management by fact, focus on results, and creating value" underpin the contemporary view on performance excellence (National Institute of Standards and Technology 2006, 1), organizations that subscribe to a political perspective of operating will likely face conflicts similar to the one just described. While managers may learn effective tactics from the political domain, a political perspective for managing the organization will limit its ability to progress along the quality continuum (see Chapter 1).

Integrating Double-Loop Learning

In one large hospital, a nursing supervisor complained to the manager of environmental services that when the housekeeper was asked to move a piece of equipment to prepare a room for a patient admission, the housekeeper refused to do so. The supervisor accused the housekeeper of being uncooperative and an obstacle to patient care. The supervisor operated from a professional mind-set and believed the housekeeper should be able to determine when the medical equipment may be touched. Because of language, cultural, and educational differences among staff in entry-level positions, the environmental services staff needed to strictly adhere to the department's standard policies and procedures. The housekeeper was operating from one set of assumptions (i.e., following the rules by not touching the nurses' equipment), while the nursing supervisor was operating from a conflicting set of assumptions (i.e., doing whatever needs to be done to care for the patient). Although both parties were trying to do their jobs the best way they knew how, their opposing assumptions led to conflict and antagonism between the two departments.

This situation of "accidental adversaries" may be unintentionally created when underlying assumptions are not known. The numerous roles, backgrounds, personalities, levels of education, and other diverse characteristics of the healthcare workforce necessitate managers to use double-loop learning as a valuable strategy to promote teamwork and quality within their scope of responsibility. Double-loop learning occurs when underlying assumptions are examined and when subsequent action, based on what the assumptions reveal, is taken (Argyris 1991). In the workplace, however, managers unfortunately often spend more time trying to mend adversarial relationships than preventing them. Managers may minimize accidental adversaries by

- clarifying operating principles,
- helping staff understand and communicate their own assumptions,

- helping staff ask for clarification and explanations of others' behavior, and
- explicitly describing their (managers') own expectations for individual employees and for teams.

Double-loop learning is not appropriate for all situations in a health services organization. For example, in the middle of an emergency resuscitation is not the time to question why a cardiac arrest code is carried out in a certain manner. As described in Chapter 1, efficiency and consistency in day-to-day operations are accomplished through minimizing variation in how processes are carried out. However, double-loop learning should be an integral part of efforts that require innovative solutions or that require improved levels of performance. Managers and teams should be comfortable with asking themselves and others questions such as, "Why do we do things the way we do? Is there a better way to get the job done? Are my own mental models helping or hurting my and our team's/department's/organization's effectiveness?"

For an improvement team, double-loop learning may take the form of discussions that question "whether operating norms are appropriate—then inventing new norms as needed" (Pierce 2000, 15). Innovative solutions (e.g., open-access scheduling) result from the process of double-loop learning. This type of scheduling approach, which is used by pediatricians and family practitioners, challenges operating norms and assumptions around outpatient scheduling (Randolph and Lannon 2001; Tumolo 2002). Managers may consider assigning a team member to be the "devil's advocate" and present an opposing view to ensure that assumptions are tested and challenged; otherwise, the challenger may be viewed as a barrier to the team process.

Conclusion

This chapter introduces the concept of systemic structure in organizations and explores lessons and strategies for managers. If managers and organizations are to achieve new levels of performance, managers must begin to integrate double-loop learning into their philosophy and approaches. The exercise at the end of this chapter provides an opportunity to explore how mental models influence behavior. Section III of this book challenges assumptions about some common management operating norms and presents a new set of norms that enhance an individual's ability to operate from a quality management perspective.

Companion Readings

Starr, P. 1982. *The Social Transformation of American Medicine: The Rise of a Sovereign Profession and the Making of a Vast Industry*, 235–89. Reading, MA: The Perseus Books Group.

Tucker, A., and A. C. Edmondson. 2003. "Why Hospitals Don't Learn from Failures: Organizational and Psychological Dynamics that Inhibit System Change." *California Management Review* 45 (2): 55–72.

References

Argyris, C. 1991. "Teaching Smart People How to Learn." *Harvard Business Review* 69 (3): 99–110.

Armenakis, A. A., and A. G. Bedian. 1992. "The Role of Metaphors in Organizational Change." *Group and Organizational Management* 17 (3): 242–48.

Cabana, M. D., C. S. Rand, N. R. Powe, A. W. Wu, M. H. Wilson, P. A. Abboud, and H. R. Rubin. 1999. "Why Don't Physicians Follow Clinical Practice Guidelines? A Framework for Improvement." *JAMA* 282 (15): 1458–65.

Clearly, C., and T. Packard. 1992. "The Use of Metaphors in Organizational Assessment and Change." *Group and Organizational Management* 17 (3): 229–41.

GLACIER. 2003. [Online information; retrieved 2/16/03]. www.glacier.rice.edu.

Gordon, S. 2005. *Nursing Against the Odds: How Health Care Cost Cutting, Media Stereotypes and Medical Hubris Undermine Nurses and Patient Care.* Ithaca, NY: Cornell University Press.

Hanna, D. P. 1988. *Designing Organizations for High Performance.* Reading, MA: Addison-Wesley Publishing Company.

Innovations Associates. 1995. "Systems Thinking: A Language for Learning and Action." Participant manual, version 95.4.1. Waltham, MA: Innovations Associates.

Institute of Medicine. 1999. *To Err Is Human: Building a Safer Health System,* edited by L. T. Kohn, J. M. Corrigan, and M. S. Donaldson. Washington, DC: National Academies Press.

———. 2001. Crossing the *Quality Chasm: A New Health System for the 21st Century.* Washington, DC: National Academies Press.

Kaiser Family Foundation, Agency for Healthcare Research and Quality, Harvard School of Public Health. 2004. "National Survey on Consumers' Experiences with Patient Safety and Quality Information." Menlo Park, CA: Kaiser Family Foundation.

Kelly, D. L. 1999. "Systems Thinking: A Tool for Organizational Diagnosis in Healthcare." In *Making It Happen: Stories from Inside the New Workplace,* compiled from The Systems Thinker Newsletter, 1989–97. Waltham, MA: Pegasus Communications.

McCormack, B., A. Kitson, G. Harvey, J. Rycroft-Malone, A. Titchen, and K. Seers. 2002. "Getting Evidence into Practice: The Meaning of 'Context'." *Journal of Advanced Nursing* 38 (1): 94–104.

McGlynn, E. A., S. M. Asch, J. Adams, J. Keesy, J. Hicks, A. DeCristofaro, and E. A. Kerr. 2003. "The Quality of Health Care Delivered to Adults in the United States." *New England Journal of Medicine* 348 (26): 2635–45.

National Institute of Standards and Technology. 2006. Baldrige National
    Quality Program Healthcare Criteria for Performance Excellence.
    [Online information; retrieved 1/2/06.] www.baldrige.gov/Criteria.htm.

Pierce, J. C. 2000. "The Paradox of Physicians and Administrators in Healthcare
    Organizations." *Healthcare Management Review* 25 (1): 7–28.

Randolph, G., and C. Lannon. 2001. "Advanced Access Scheduling: Doing
    Today's Work Today." *American Academy of Pediatrics News* 19 (6): 266.

Senge, P. M. 1990. *The Fifth Discipline: The Art and Practice of the Learning
    Organization.* New York: Doubleday Currency.

Shortell, S. M., and A. D. Kaluzny. 2000. *Healthcare Management: Organization
    Design and Behavior.* Albany, NY: Delmar Thomson Learning.

Shortell, S. M., J. L. O'Brien, J. M. Carman, R. W. Foster, E. F. X. Hughes, H.
    Boerstler, and E. J. O'Connor. 1995. "Assessing the Impact of
    Continuous Quality Improvement/Total Quality Management: Concept
    versus Implementation." *Healthcare Research* 30 (2): 377–99.

Solberg, L. I. 2000a. "Incentivising, Facilitating and Implementing an Office
    Tobacco Cessation System." *Tobacco Control* 9 (Suppl 1): i37–41.

———. 2000b. "Lessons from Experienced Guideline Implementers: Attend to
    Many Factors and Use Multiple Strategies." *Joint Commission Journal on
    Quality Improvement* 26 (4): 171–88.

———. 2002. "Guideline Implementation: Why Don't We Do It?" *American
    Family Physician* 65 (2): 176, 181–82.

Starr, P. 1982. *The Social Transformation of American Medicine: The Rise of a
    Sovereign Profession and the Making of a Vast Industry.* Reading, MA: The
    Perseus Books Group.

Tumolo, J. 2002. "Open-Access Scheduling." *Advanced Nurse Practitioner* 10
    (5): 25.

Weisbord, M. R. 1987. *Productive Workplaces: Organizing and Managing for
    Dignity and Community.* San Francisco: Jossey-Bass.

Exercise

Objective: To practice identifying underlying structures and determining how mental models or assumptions influence behavior in organizations.

Instructions

1. This chapter discussed the iceberg as a metaphor for gaining a deeper understanding of a system. The chapter also discussed the need to ask not only the question, "What can we *do* differently?" but also, "How can we best understand why we are getting the results we are getting?" The Institute of Medicine's (IOM) report, *Crossing the Quality Chasm: A New Health System for the 21st Century,* recommends ten new rules for redesigning healthcare processes. These rules may be thought of as replies to the question, "What can we *do* differently?" In the Underlying Structures Worksheet below,

the first column contains four of the IOM rules. The middle column contains the current state of the U.S. healthcare system relative to the rule (readers will recognize some of these statements from Figure 1.1). Complete the third column of the worksheet by answering the question, What underlying structures are contributing to the current state? Write your responses on the worksheet.

Underlying Structures Worksheet

Redesigned Rule (IOM 2001)	Current State of the Healthcare System	What underlying structures contribute to this system behavior in the United States?
Care based on continuous healing relationship	Fragmentation across payers, providers, geographic locations	
The patient as the source of control	Fifty-five percent of Americans surveyed are dissatisfied with the quality of healthcare in the United States, and 40 percent responded that in the past five years, quality of care has gotten worse (Kaiser Family Foundation 2004)	
Evidence-based decision making	Adult Americans received 54.9 percent of recommended preventive care, acute care, and chronic care (McGlynn et al. 2003)	
Safety as a system property	Between 44,000 and 98,000 deaths per year in the United States have been attributed to preventable medical errors, making medical errors the eighth leading cause of death (IOM 1999)	

2. a. See the Mental Models Worksheet below. Identify two different mental models associated with the "fighting fires" management style in the context of a healthcare organization. Write your responses in the respective boxes on the worksheet.

    b. Describe how each of these mental models would influence your actions and behavior in your role as a healthcare manager. Write your response in the respective boxes on the worksheet.

    c. Choose the mental model that currently influences you or that you would like to influence your management approach and style. Circle that mental model on the worksheet.

Mental Models Worksheet

	Mental Model	Actions	Alternative Mental Model	Actions
"Fighting fires" management style				

ACHIEVING QUALITY RESULTS IN COMPLEX SYSTEMS

GOALS

Objectives

- To explore why effective goal setting is essential to quality management
- To gain an appreciation for the relationship between how goals are stated and the ability to obtain desired results
- To contrast different types of goal statements
- To practice setting goals

A guest lecturer, formerly a neonatal intensive care nurse, leads health administration doctoral students on a discussion about organizational effectiveness. At the conclusion of the discussion, one student observes that the previous guest lecturer also had a background in pediatrics (Bordley et al. 2001; Margolis et al. 2001). The student asks the lecturer if there is a relationship between an interest in quality and a background in pediatrics. The guest lecturer pauses for reflection and then replies, "Maybe it's because we see life at its beginning and understand how important a healthy start to life is."

The same idea can be applied to the setting of goals. A "healthy start" to an improvement effort or management intervention begins with an effective goal. This chapter explores the reason that effective goal setting is essential to quality management, the relationship between goals and results, and the approaches that managers can employ to improve their goal-setting skills.

Importance of Setting Goals

In healthcare organizations, the influence of goals on quality may be seen in both clinical interventions and management interventions.

Clinical Interventions

Patient A presents to his primary care provider as overweight and suffering from high blood pressure. The treatment goals the provider sets for the patient are to lose weight and to take the prescribed blood pressure medicine. The patient begins dieting and taking his blood pressure medicine. Within six months, Patient A has lost 30 pounds and shows improved blood pressure.

However, at Patient A's annual checkup several months later, his provider is dismayed to find that he has gained back the 30 pounds.

Patient B is also overweight and suffering from high blood pressure when she sees her primary care provider. The treatment goals the provider sets for the patient are to integrate a balanced diet and regular exercise into her daily lifestyle and to reduce blood pressure through lifestyle change and medication. Within six months, Patient B has also lost 30 pounds and shows improved blood pressure. At her next annual physical, Patient B has kept off the 30 pounds and informs her provider that she feels much better as she has been walking three days a week and eating healthier.

The seemingly subtle difference in how the treatment goals were set for these two patients actually represents the relationship between the goals and the subsequent results that are obtained. Patient A and Patient B both presented with similar situations. Both providers were conscientious and caring and made the appropriate diagnosis. The difference in the impact and sustainability of the interventions was in how the goals were set.

Managerial Interventions

Goals serve many purposes in organizations (Scott 1998); they are integrated into most aspects of a manager's role and functions at all levels of the organization. Goals help a manager to select among many alternative courses of action. For example, for the goal of improving patient satisfaction by reducing waiting times in the clinic, a proposed intervention that would reduce waiting times but would be perceived negatively by patients would be disregarded, while a proposed intervention that would reduce waiting times but would be perceived as patient friendly would be considered.

Goals are used to provide direction for decision making. An organizational goal to increase market share in obstetrics influences management decisions when faced with prioritizing capital expenditures for remodeling patient care units in the hospital. An organizational goal of being the first-choice medical provider in the community may serve to motivate employees and other stakeholders. A goal of "becoming a role model in patient-centered care" may be used to promote an ideology or philosophy of care, such as the Planetree (2003) philosophy. A goal to become a "center of excellence" for cardiovascular care may foster employee pride and loyalty, serve as a recruitment strategy for physicians and other clinical providers, and bring prestige within the community. A goal to be the "premier center for cancer research" can legitimize investment in research infrastructure at an academic medical center; successful research, in turn, will position the center well to acquire additional research funding

When used in conjunction with performance measurement, goals determine whether the data demonstrate favorable or unfavorable organizational performance. In the absence of a goal or a measure, it is difficult to hold people accountable for improving performance or maintaining required competencies.

When managers realize how pervasively goals are used within clinical and organizational settings, they may begin to appreciate the widespread impact of effective goal-setting skills on organizational performance. The importance of setting effective goals may be further appreciated when one realizes that all subsequent actions follow and are influenced by how the initial goal is set.

Relationship Between Goals and Results

The ability to set goals effectively is a requisite skill for managers at all levels of an organization. The following example of two hospitals facing a similar challenge illustrates how goals set by leadership influence subsequent actions and the results of those actions.

Hospital A and Hospital B both use a national vendor to measure and report patient satisfaction. The reports show that both hospitals perform below the national average for hospitals of a similar size and type. Senior leaders at each hospital decided to focus on improving customer service and patient satisfaction as an organizational priority. To address the problem of low patient satisfaction, the senior management team at Hospital A set the following goal: improve customer service.

To achieve this goal, Hospital A hired a customer service specialist and instituted mandatory customer service training for all employees. The nurse managers in the hospital were then faced with a dilemma. Their department education budgets were limited, and their staff were already subject to mandatory education in areas such as infection control and fire safety. One more mandatory educational requirement would deplete the education dollars and eliminate the managers' resources for funding continuing education to maintain the staff's clinical competence.

When a goal offers little direction and is very vague, like Hospital A's goal, the result is often an approach to a type of problem solving called "repair service behavior," where organizations or individuals solve a "problem" they know how to solve, whether or not it is the problem they need to solve (Dorner 1996). An example of repair service behavior is when a novice gardener responds to the problem of withering leaves on a new plant by watering the plant more instead of repotting and fertilizing, which are what the plant needs.

Hospital A knew how to create new positions and conduct training. However, it did not know how to identify the underlying cause of a widespread organizational problem. This example also illustrates how a poorly conceived goal (improve customer service) is likely to cause unintended consequences or even more problems in other areas of the organization. In this case, the mandatory customer-service training took resources away from technical education and over time risked reducing the overall technical competency of the nursing staff.

Hospital B used a different approach to address the problem of low patient satisfaction. Because the source of the problem was not evident to

Hospital B's administrators, they needed to first gain a better understanding of why the problem was occurring before making a decision on specific interventions. The senior management team at Hospital B set the following partial or intermediate goal: identify contributing factors to patient dissatisfaction. This goal guided further study of the hospital's satisfaction data, which showed that patients were most dissatisfied by lack of communication with nurses and with patient preparation for discharge. The organization conducted a root-cause analysis to learn why communication and discharge planning were not occurring effectively. The analysis revealed that, although staffing seemed adequate on a day-to-day basis, the hospital's reliance on temporary staff and traveling nurses had increased significantly over the past year. Although the temporary staff and traveling nurses were experienced in their technical duties, their lack of familiarity with the hospital's specific procedures and resources increasingly led to communication breakdowns both within and among departments. The organizational analysis highlighted this common problem for the departments responsible for patient registration, billing, and housekeeping as well as in the nursing, respiratory therapy, and pharmacy departments. On the basis of this information, senior leaders at Hospital B could then prioritize the contributing factors and develop specific goals to address the top-priority contributing factors. They revised their goals as follows: (1) increase the proportion of staff who are permanent employees, (2) improve the discharge planning process, (2) reallocate resources spent on temporary staff to fund the aforementioned improvements, and (4) monitor the impact of staffing and process improvements on patient satisfaction.

The process Hospital B used illustrates the senior leaders' understanding of how goal setting should be approached in complex systems such as healthcare organizations (Dorner 1996, 63–64):

- When working with a complex, dynamic system, we must first develop at least a provisional picture of the partial goals we want to achieve; those partial goals will clarify what we need to do when.
- In complex situations, we must almost always avoid focusing on just one element and pursuing only one goal; instead, we must pursue several goals at once.

By approaching the problem using a partial goal, Hospital B avoided an intervention that may not have solved the problem, and it was able to avoid the repair service behavior often associated with an unclear goal. Instead, once Hospital B defined the underlying problems a clear, multiple-goal statement was set to guide the improvement interventions.

Chapter 5 discusses latent management errors and their role in medical errors. Each of the sources of management errors described in Chapter 5, "inadequate preparation of/by decision maker(s), political pressure, flawed decision-maker process, and ignorance of legitimate alternatives" (Hofmann 2005, 11) imply faulty goal setting within an organization's management or administrative domain. By improving their goal-setting skills, managers may decrease their contribution to latent management errors and, in turn, improve patient safety in their organizations.

Approaches to Setting Goals

This section is not intended to teach managers how to do strategic planning. Rather, the intent is to provide managers with approaches that, once appropriate data are collected and preliminary problems are identified, they may use to help them set effective goals for their own departments and organizations.

Use Intermediate Goals

Although vague, general, or unclear goals may lead to repair service behavior, phrasing a partial goal in general terms is useful to set the overall direction (as illustrated in the previous example). Specific goals can be established once decision makers gain new information and clarity about the problem. For example, a surgical services manager may use general goals to set the overall direction for his department over the next several years. These goals may be to improve clinical outcomes, improve patient satisfaction, improve cost effectiveness, and integrate services across multiple sites. Each year, during the annual planning process, specific short-term or intermediate goals may also be established. The goal in Year 1 may be to implement a standard performance measurement system across all sites. The goal in Year 2 may be to increase the percentage of first surgical cases for the day that are started on time for each of the operating rooms in the service. The goal in Year 3 may be to implement standard preoperative testing protocols to eliminate unnecessary variation in preoperative tests (Kelly et al. 1997).

In this example, a general goal is used to communicate overall direction. Because the manager also understands the concept and importance of partial goals, he is able to establish the first partial goal (measurement system) to help him understand how to prioritize subsequent annual improvement goals.

Define Implicit Goals

The surgical services manager in the example above also understands the concept of implicit goals—that is, a goal that may be intuitive but not necessarily purposefully addressed. For example, the manager knows that to achieve the desired level of performance, cultivating positive and collaborative relationships between physicians and administrators is essential. Although not explicitly defined in the manager's other performance goals, this implicit goal guides the approaches that the manager selected for designing the performance measurement system and for improving first-case start times. As a result of the manager's implicit goal of building relationships in Years 1 and 2, implementing a clinical standard of care can be accomplished more smoothly in Year 3, which may not be possible without the benefit of improved working relationships between physicians and administrators.

Whenever possible, managers should try to identify implicit goals so they may be defined and communicated and an "accidental adversaries" situation (described in the previous chapter) may be avoided.

Reformulate Goals As Needed

Managers may find that setting goals is an iterative process; that is, as new information becomes available, managers must be willing to evaluate previous goals and reformulate goals as needed. For example, a nurse manager of a 30-bed, medical-surgical patient unit was faced with improving the overall performance of her unit. Because the unit was the major inpatient unit of a small community hospital, she was faced with a major overhaul rather than simply a single improvement. However, she also realized that the goal of "overhaul performance" was too vague to identify specific interventions, expectations, and action plans for her staff.

She reformulated her original goal—"overhaul performance"—to more clearly establish the general direction of the performance improvement effort. Her new goals were as follows: (1) promote teamwork, (2) promote continuity of care, (3) meet or exceed local and national standards of care, (4) integrate performance improvement into the daily work environment, (5) promote staff satisfaction, and (6) improve cost effectiveness.

Set Multiple Goals

The nurse manager in the previous example demonstrated another important approach for setting effective goals. Because of the interrelationships among activities, processes, and other elements in healthcare organizations, managers will find that focusing on multiple interrelated goals is necessary. Although a single goal may be useful for a simple process improvement, a systems perspective suggests the need for setting multiple goals that may be carried out concurrently and/or sequentially to take into account the interrelationships within the system. The systems models in Chapter 5 may guide managers in identifying areas for consideration when establishing multiple goals.

In this medical-surgical unit, the nurse manager assembled a team of charge nurses to work together intensively for a series of meetings to help determine how to meet the unit's goals. After several meetings directed toward understanding the hospital's history, operating requirements, and environmental challenges; analyzing current processes; and identifying causes of performance gaps, the team discussed its ideal vision for the unit. They described their ideal unit according to desired clinical outcomes, the nature of their relationships with patients and families, teamwork, and business requirements. This vision became the unit's long-term goal.

The members of the team realized that, to achieve this multifaceted vision, they must also focus on multiple interdependent interventions. They also realized that, although they would not be able to implement multiple interventions all at once because of resource constraints, it was important to identify, prioritize, and establish timelines for the multiple goals; this would serve as the "road map" of their vision. The team found that some of the interventions (e.g., establishing a staff communication book and bulletin board) could be implemented immediately without much effort. The team realized that some of the goals (e.g., improving the way in which daily census and productivity were tracked, reported, communicated, and managed) would take a month or so to implement and were identified as short-term goals. The team learned that some of the goals (e.g., clarifying care-team roles, structure, and job descriptions) required more in-depth development and implementation considerations and were identified as medium-term goals.

The team converted an implicit goal to an explicit one when it established the following long-term goal: enhance the personal accountability of all staff. Clear goals provided the direction, while a performance measurement system and a simple project-tracking report enabled the manager, the team, and the unit staff to track their progress toward their goals and their progress toward becoming their ideal unit.

Types of Goal Statements

Along with understanding the various approaches used in setting effective goals, managers must purposefully craft a goal statement that will best help them succeed in a given situation. For example, a manager has just learned that the immunization rates for the patients in his large pediatric practice are below both the state and national averages. He is faced with the problem of substandard immunization rates. How does he now communicate improvement goals to the practice in ways that will enable him to utilize the approaches just described?

Some types of goal statements have been introduced through the examples presented earlier in the chapter. The different types of goals may be thought of as pairs of opposites: positive or negative, general or specific, clear or unclear, simple or multiple, and implicit or explicit (Dorner 1996). Table 8.1 provides a definition for each of these types and examples of how each may be used by the manager of the pediatric practice.

When faced with a problem to solve, managers may state their goal in different ways and evaluate the pros and cons of each statement as a way to enhance their decision-making skills. Consider the following situation. The medical director of an emergency department for a large, acute care hospital has just reviewed the department's quality indicators that will be

TABLE 8.1
Examples of Goals

Definition	Type of Goal	Example
Working toward a desired condition versus making an undesirable condition go away	Positive	Achieve immunization rates that are in the top 10 percent statewide.
	Negative	Reduce the number of patients with incomplete immunizations.
Few criteria versus multiple criteria	General	Improve immunization rates.
	Specific	Ensure all infants in the practice receive the appropriate vaccinations at ages 1 month, 2 months, 4 months, 6 months, 12 months, 15 months, 18 months, and 24 months according to the Centers for Disease Control and Prevention Recommended Childhood Immunization Schedule.
Difficult to determine if the goal has been met versus precise criteria permitting the evaluation of whether the goal is being met	Unclear	Work with the office staff to improve pediatric care.
	Clear	Our clinic will select a team to enroll in the quality improvement course offered by the State Pediatric Association from April through September. The team will design and implement processes to improve the clinic's compliance with the Recommended Childhood Immunization Schedule. The team will measure overall immunization rates on a quarterly basis. Results will be reported at staff meetings.
Single goal versus series of sequential or concurrent goals that take into account relationships within the system	Simple	Give age-appropriate immunizations at each well-child appointment.
	Multiple	Track patient compliance with well-child exams. Notify and schedule patients who have missed well-child exams. Give age-appropriate immunizations during well-child exams.
Obvious versus hidden	Implicit	Improve immunization rates.
	Explicit	Improve the ability to identify, deliver, and monitor pediatric preventative care services, including age-appropriate immunizations.

Source: Data from Dorner, D. 1996. *The Logic of Failure: Recognizing and Avoiding Error in Complex Situations.* Reading, MA: Perseus Books.

published on Medicare's Hospital Compare website (see Chapter 6). The hospital's performance on the indicators for care of patients with acute myocardial infarction (AMI) is below the average performance of all hospitals in the state. The administrator for emergency services has asked for a plan to improve hospital performance in the following areas (Jencks, Huff, and Cuerdon 2003):

- Timeliness of administration of aspirin
- Prescribing aspirin at discharge
- Smoking-cessation counseling

The medical director uses a chart like the one shown in Table 8.2 to evaluate the options for the improvement goal.

Upon reviewing the goal options, that medical director reviews her findings with the administrator. "This is an odd scenario. The only item for a patient who is suffering from an AMI that would be handled in an emergency department is appropriate timing of the aspirin administration. Smoking cessation counseling and discharge medications would be handled on discharge from the cardiology service. No patient with AMI would be discharged from the emergency department. The ultimate goal statement combines desirable qualities from several types. I choose the following positive and specific goal statements:

- Improve the proportion of patients with suspected AMI who receive ASA within the first 5 minutes of arrival to 90 percent or more. (Or greater than the statewide average.)
- Improve the number of patients with AMI who receive a prescription for ASA on discharge to 100 percent.
- Improve the number of smokers with AMI who receive smoking cessation counseling before discharge to 100 percent.

The language of the goal statements conveys a positive approach. Specific targets indicate the specific nature of the improvement effort. Much of goals 2 and 3 can be implemented through preprinted order sheets that are signed on admission" (Nissman 2005).

Through the process of evaluating the pros and cons of possible goal statements, the medical director and the administrator were guided to address the larger issues of how the organization incorporates, documents, and measures evidence-based care in a consistent manner for this patient population along the entire continuum of care from admission to discharge. Rather than implementing the quick fix of having a case manager "nag" physicians in the emergency department and again before the patient's discharge as most hospitals in the area were doing, the medical director's approach to setting performance improvement goals promoted a more systemic solution to improve outcomes for AMI patients while fulfilling Medicare requirements. In addition, the goals served to improve outcomes for all patients with AMI, not simply the subset of patients who met the Hospital Compare inclusion criteria.

TABLE 8.2
Goal Statement Options

Type of Goal	Goal Statements	Pros	Cons
Positive	Increase number of patients with acute myocardial infarction who receive aspirin at presentation and discharge to exceed statewide averages. Increase the number of smokers presenting with acute myocardial infarction who are offered smoking-cessation counseling to exceed statewide averages.	Engenders a positive atmosphere and provides a goal to achieve rather than implying one is sub par	Not all people are motivated by positive goals; might be considered optional
Negative	Reduce the number of patients receiving aspirin beyond the statewide average time. Reduce the number of patients not being prescribed aspirin at discharge. Reduce number of smokers with acute myocardial infarction who leave the hospital without smoking-cessation counseling.	Implies a deficiency that needs to be corrected (or else)	Many people don't respond well to negativity
General	Increase the number of patients with acute myocardial infarction who receive aspirin in a timely manner. Increase the number of patients with acute myocardial infarction who receive a prescription for aspirin at discharge. Increase the number of patients with acute myocardial infarction who receive smoking-cessation counseling before discharge.	Conveys broad intent of the problem to be solved	Not very practical; difficult to measure
Specific	Ensure that all patients presenting with possible acute myocardial infarction receive aspirin within 5 minutes of arrival to the emergency department. Ensure that all patients with acute myocardial infarction receive a prescription for aspirin on discharge. Ensure that all smokers with acute myocardial infarction receive smoking-cessation counseling before discharge.	Has the danger of missing the forest for the trees	Very practical and measurable

Source: Data from D. Nissman. 2005. Used with permission.

Conclusion

Effective goals precede effective performance. This chapter has explored approaches that managers may use to improve their own goal-setting skills. Although there is no single correct or incorrect approach to setting a goal, managers should be aware of the advantages and pitfalls of each approach and the ways the goals are communicated. The exercise at the end of this chapter provides an opportunity to set goals in different ways, to critique the alternative goals, and to select the most appropriate and effective goal. Chapter 9 explores assumptions around another management norm: purpose. Often expressed as an organizational or departmental mission statement, a clear understanding and definition of purpose may be considered a high-leverage systemic structure.

Companion Readings

Dorner, D. 1996. *The Logic of Failure: Recognizing and Avoiding Error in Complex Situations*, 49–70. Reading, MA: Perseus Books.

Klein, G., and K. E. Weick. 2000. "Decisions: Making the Right Ones, Learning from the Wrong Ones." *Across the Board* 37 (6): 16–22. Available online: www.conference-board.org/articles/atb_article.cfm?id=96.

References

Bordley, W. C., P. A. Margolis, J. Stuart, C. Lannon, and L. Keyes. 2001. "Improving Preventive Service Delivery Through Office Systems." *Pediatrics* 108 (3): E41.

Dorner, D. 1996. *The Logic of Failure: Recognizing and Avoiding Error in Complex Situations*. Reading, MA: Perseus Books.

Hofmann, P. B. 2005. "Acknowledging and Examining Management Mistakes." In *Management Mistakes in Healthcare: Identification, Correction and Prevention*, edited by P. B. Hofmann and F. Perry, 3-27. Cambridge, UK: Cambridge University Press.

Hospital Compare website. www.hospitalcompare.hhs.gov/Hospital/Static /Data-Professionals.asp?dest=NAV|Home|DataDetails |ProfessionalInfo#measureset.

Jencks, S. F., E. D. Huff, and T. Cuerdon. 2003. "Change in the Quality of Care Delivered to Medicare Beneficiaries, 1998–1999 to 2000–2001." *JAMA* 289 (3): 305–12.

Jha, A. K., Z. Li, E. J. Orav, and A. M. Epstein. 2005. "Care in U.S. Hospitals—The Hospital Quality Alliance Program." *New England Journal of Medicine* 353 (3): 265–74.

Kelly, D. L., S. L. Pestotnik, M. C. Coons, and J. W. Lelis. 1997. "Reengineering a Surgical Service Line: Focusing on Core Process Improvement." *American Journal of Medical Quality* 12 (2): 120–29.

Margolis, P. A., R. Stevens, W. C. Bordley, J. Stuart, C. Harlan, L. Keyes-Elstein, and S. Wisseh. 2001. "From Concept to Application: The Impact of a Community-wide Intervention to Improve the Delivery of Preventive Services to Children." *Pediatrics* 108 (3): E42.

Nissman, D. 2005. Excerpt from an unpublished document.

Planetree. 2003. [Online information; retrieved 2/18/03.] www.planetree.org/.

Scott, W. R. 1998. *Organizations: Rational, Natural and Open Systems*. Upper Saddle River, NJ: Prentice Hall.

Exercise

Objective: To practice linking goal statements with results.

Instructions

1. The original set of Medicare Hospital Quality Measures have grown and been refined over time (Jencks, Huff, and Cuerdon 2003; Jha et al. 2005). At the end of 2005, CMS defined the following hospital quality measures (see www.hospitalcompare.hhs.gov):

    Acute myocardial infarction
    *   Percent of patients given angiotensin-converting enzyme inhibitor for left ventricular dysfunction
    *   Percent of patients given adult smoking-cessation advice/counseling
    *   Percent of patients given aspirin at arrival
    *   Percent of patients given aspirin at discharge
    *   Percent of patients given beta blocker at arrival
    *   Percent of patients given beta blocker at discharge
    *   Percent of patients give percutaneous coronary intervention within 120 minutes of arrival
    *   Percent of patients given thrombolytic medication within 30 minutes of arrival

    Congestive heart failure
    *   Percent of patients given angiotensin-converting enzyme inhibitor for left ventricular dysfunction
    *   Percent of patients given adult smoking-cessation advice/counseling
    *   Percent of patients given assessment of left ventricular function
    *   Percent of patients given discharge instructions

    Community-acquired pneumonia
    *   Percent of patients assessed and given pneumococcal vaccination
    *   Percent of patients given adult smoking-cessation advice/counseling

- Percent of patients given initial antibiotic(s) within four hours after arrival
- Percent of patients given oxygenation assessment
- Percent of patients given the most appropriate antibiotic(s)
- Percent of patients having a blood culture performed prior to first antibiotic received in the hospital

Surgical quality measures

- Percent of surgery patients who received preventive antibiotic(s) one hour before incision
- Percent of surgery patients whose preventive antibiotics are stopped within 24 hours after surgery

2. Read the following study results:

> Analysis of data from the Hospital Quality Alliance national reporting system shows that performance varies among hospitals and across indicators.... [P]erformance scores for acute myocardial infarction closely predicted performance scores for congestive health failure but not for pneumonia.... [O]ur findings indicate that quality measures had only moderate predictive ability across the three conditions. Although a high quality of care for acute myocardial infarction predicted a high quality of care for congestive heart failure, the former was only marginally better than chance for identifying a high quality of care for pneumonia. These data do not provide support for the notion that 'good' hospitals are easy to identify or consistent in their performance across conditions (Jha et al. 2005, 265, 272).

Write one sentence that summarizes these results. Describe your insights into how organizational goals may have contributed to achieving these results.

3. Define and write the problem(s) illustrated in the study by Jha and colleagues. Practice your goal-setting skills by writing three possible goals to address the problem(s).

4. Critique the three goal statements, and document your critique on a worksheet such as the one below.

Goals Worksheet

Goal Statement	Type of Goal	Pros	Cons

5. Select your preferred goal statement. Describe your rationale for selecting this statement.

PURPOSE

Objectives

- To explore the importance of purpose to quality management
- To gain an appreciation for the role of purpose in obtaining desired results
- To describe an approach for clarifying purpose
- To practice using the purpose principle

The quality department at Hospital A defines its mission as "Helping departments improve their quality indicators to meet regulatory requirements." The hospital has consistently met the JCAHO performance requirements and has demonstrated improvement on the clinical indicators for Medicare beneficiaries required by CMS (Jencks, Huff, and Cuerdon 2003). However, physicians at Hospital A consistently complain to the CEO about bottlenecks in scheduling x-ray examinations for their patients and delays in receiving results for just about any diagnostic test.

The quality department at Hospital B defines its mission as "Providing technical and consultative support to departments, managers, and teams to help them improve value to their customers." Hospital B also consistently meets the JCAHO performance requirements and demonstrates improvement in the CMS clinical indicators. However, Hospital B also demonstrates improved cycle times in numerous clinical diagnostic processes and has reduced its overall operational costs and improved employee satisfaction and retention.

Organizations and departments often use a mission statement to define their identity—that is, to explain why the organization or department exists, what the department is organized to do, or what a group is trying to achieve. In this book, the identity or reason for being is referred to as *purpose*. Just as subsequent actions are influenced by the way a goal is defined, actions are also influenced by the way a purpose is defined. While there is some overlap in the concepts of goals and purpose, in this book, the term "goal" refers to a desired end and the term "purpose" refers to a group's reason for being. Understanding and effectively using purpose and goals go hand in hand when viewing quality management from a systems perspective. Managers often face the need to reevaluate, revise, and redefine the initial goals based on their deeper understanding of the purpose of an initiative. In this way, purpose can be a tool to help managers reformulate partial or general goals as they gather more information about the problem.

The quality department in Hospital A defined itself in terms of a single goal rather than a purpose; the department was looking to attain specific results in accordance with defined performance indicators. Hospital A succeeded in achieving these results, but it was not successful in achieving an overall quality organization. In Hospital B, the quality department defined itself as a resource to others in the hospital to help improve the value of services provided. One of the goals of the quality department in this instance could have been to improve care delivered to those patient populations addressed by the indicators. By improving the hospital's overall discharge process, for example, the department improved not only the ability to identify patients at risk for pneumonia and administer pneumococcal and influenza immunizations before discharge (required indicators) but also the overall quality of the patient and family's transition from the acute care setting to home, home care, or long-term care (Jencks, Huff, and Cuerdon 2003).

Managers should consciously and consistently question purpose at all levels of the organization—that is, the purpose of individual activities, jobs/roles, processes, departments, and the organization overall. A clear understanding of purpose guides managers in establishing direction for improvements, helps managers to know they are working on the right problems, and increases the likelihood that quality efforts will achieve intended results. Without a clear understanding of purpose, managers run the risk of wasting time and resources by working on the wrong problem or even improving something that should not exist in the first place.

This chapter explores the concept of purpose and its importance for managers. Approaches that managers may use to define, refine, and clarify purpose are also discussed.

The Importance of Purpose

In Chapter 1, Donabedian's causal relationship of quality-of-care measures was described as Structure ➡ Process ➡ Outcome. However, when designing or redesigning interventions to improve results, the sequence is conceptually reversed: a clear understanding of purpose should guide the way organizations define desired outcomes. The purpose and desired outcomes should guide the way processes are designed to support achieving that purpose, and the structure (how people are organized, roles are defined, and tools and technology are selected) should be guided by the requirements of the process. This sequence may be thought of as Purpose/Desired Outcomes ➡ Process ➡ Structure.

When using this conceptual sequence, understanding and clarifying purpose serve an important role in setting direction and ensuring that the right problem is being addressed. Discussions of purpose can also foster common ground and promote breakthrough ideas and solutions.

Setting Direction

A student's purpose or identity shapes his selection of classes. A student with an identity of musician may take music theory and instrument classes, whereas a medical student may choose anatomy and physiology classes. Similarly, the identity of an organization or department shapes its management's choices of goals, priorities, resource allocation, and improvement targets.

A hospital-based laboratory performed tests for the inpatient and outpatient populations of the tertiary care hospital in which it was located and for smaller hospitals and physicians' offices in the area. The manager and medical director, faced with the need to redesign the laboratory's operations, set a departmental goal to redesign the processes and the work area to improve efficiency and better meet customer needs. To accomplish this they created a redesign team.

One of the first topics the redesign team discussed was the laboratory's purpose. Initially, the team described the laboratory's purpose as providing customer service. For a hospital that had formally adopted a total quality philosophy several years previously, the team's focus on customer service indicated that they had integrated this total quality principle into their way of operating. However, to provide customer service was not a reason to exist; customer service was a part of what the laboratory provided but not its sole function. It was necessary to provide something other than customer service.

The redesign facilitator and the manager invited panels of internal customers to talk with the team about their own expectations and experiences as customers of this laboratory's service. The common theme heard from each customer, whether a nurse in the emergency department or a doctor's office, was that they depended on the information the laboratory gave them to make patient care decisions. In their efforts to provide quality service, the laboratory had lost sight of the reason it existed: to provide information. The team realized that quality service was a desired characteristic in how they delivered the information.

As the team continued to discuss the laboratory's purpose, the team also realized that they provided customers with three distinct types of information. The first type of information was clinical patient data in the form of test results. Within this "product line" were numerous types of results from many types of specimens, from blood for analyzing cholesterol levels to tissue for analyzing a cancerous tumor. Over the years, however, the laboratory's role had evolved in response to changing reimbursement schemes, new technology, and published research on clinical treatments and interventions. As a result, the laboratory found itself providing its customers with two additional "product lines": (1) information in the form of technical expertise to other providers about how to use and interpret the new tests as they became available and (2) information related to the technical and regulatory requirements as more tests moved away from the laboratory to point-of-care techniques carried out by nurses or physicians.

Clarifying its purpose became an empowering realization for the laboratory staff. Each of the three product lines of information was necessary to provide laboratory services to all of its customers; however, only one—clinical laboratory results—was a potential source of measurable revenue or expense for this department; the other two product lines were solely a source of expense for the department. Equipped with a clear definition of purpose and arguing with a systems point of view, the laboratory manager and medical director were able to negotiate budgetary expectations with their administrator. They were able to articulate that the laboratory may be incurring expenses that ultimately benefited the quality of patient care in other departments and/or reduced the cost of the patient's total hospital experience. The budget discussions changed from focusing exclusively on reducing laboratory expenses to including how to measure and preserve the laboratory's essential role in providing overall quality of laboratory services to all patients within its service domain, not simply for work carried out within the boundaries of the laboratory's walls (Kelly 1998).

Addressing the Right Problem

The manager in an ambulatory surgery unit was faced with the problem of frequent patient delays that led to patient complaints and higher costs as a result of excessive length of stay. The manager assembled a team to address the goal of redesigning patient flow to improve clinical outcomes, patient satisfaction, and cost effectiveness (Kelly et al. 1997).

In one of the first redesign meetings, the facilitator asked the team to identify the major phases of care that make up the entire process of care for a patient experiencing ambulatory surgery. The team identified five phases that an ambulatory surgery patient goes through: (1) the prehospital phase—that is, care occurring somewhere other than in the ambulatory surgery unit; (2) the preoperative phase—that is, care occurring in the ambulatory surgery unit before the patient goes to the operating room; (3) the intraoperative phase—that is, the actual operation taking place in the operating room; (4) the postoperative phase—that is, care supporting patient recovery and taking place in the recovery room or the ambulatory surgery unit; and (5) the posthospitalization phase—that is, care occurring after the patient is discharged from the ambulatory surgery unit; this may include a follow-up phone call by a nurse or follow-up care in the physician's office.

The facilitator then asked the team to select an area that, if improved, could have the most impact on improving patient flow and reducing delays. The team chose the prehospital phase because this process was "upstream" to all of the others. If delays or breakdowns occurred during this phase of care, the rest of the process would also be delayed.

Next, the facilitator led a discussion about the purpose of the pre-hospital phase of care. Immediately the team replied, "To prepare the patient for surgery; to make sure the patient is ready." As the purpose discussion continued, the team had a breakthrough when they realized that, although the prehospital phase of care helped to prepare the patient, its primary purpose was to prepare the hospital to receive and care for the patient in the most effective and efficient manner. If this occurred, the patient was more likely to progress through the other phases of care without unnecessary delays or surprises. This realization of purpose, along with the understanding of the interconnectedness of operational and clinical processes (see the three core process model section in Chapter 5), played an important role in redesigning the patient-flow process.

Other efforts to redesign the patient preregistration process within the organization achieved just that—a reengineered preregistration process. An understanding of the purpose of the prehospital phase of care led the surgery team to look at preregistration in a different way. The team identified an entire package of information required before a patient's admission that helped to prepare the care providers and the facility to most efficiently provide the service of outpatient surgery. This package included not only registration information (e.g., patient demographics, insurance data) but also patient education materials, clinical preparation of the patient (e.g., laboratory results, special orders, patient history), surgery scheduling, and information about the surgical procedure so that any special equipment or supplies could be arranged for in advance. A preadmission information-gathering process was then designed to promote assembling this package of information during a patient encounter at the physician's office and making sure that the information package had arrived at the hospital in advance of the patient's admission. A phone call to the patient the day before surgery confirmed last-minute details and provided the patient with an opportunity to ask any additional questions. In this way, the facility and care providers were better prepared to receive the patient, provide individualized care, anticipate and prevent delays or cancellations as a result of miscommunication or lack of information, and decrease the preoperative length of stay (Kelly et al. 1997). While this approach to ambulatory surgery may be commonplace today, an initial reevaluation of purpose (explicitly or intuitively) has influenced the contemporary standard of care.

Fostering Common Ground

Without a clear understanding of what has to be accomplished, discussions on alternative solutions to a problem may often lead to impasses. Selecting one approach over another is hindered because people often bring to the discussion their own intense ownership of a particular solution, intervention, or idea. Discussing purpose can be a less threatening way to begin a discussion about a problem. Rather than highlighting differences among possible options and inviting comments on their perceived merit or short-comings, discussing purpose helps to create a common ground with which to focus people with divergent opinions and views.

Information systems are used in healthcare organizations for a variety of purposes: storing, retrieving, and streamlining and automating access to data. Many information systems began as accounting systems. As more clinical applications are being developed and demands for electronic medical records and computerized physician order entry increase, questioning the purpose of these systems is important to ensure that the purpose, applications, uses, and outcomes are all aligned.

The phrase "clinical decision support" is commonplace in contemporary discussions about healthcare information systems. Reviewing early efforts in designing electronic clinical-decision-support tools, however, provides insights about the role of purpose in enhancing successful implementation of new technology. The clinical epidemiology and medical informatics team at LDS Hospital in Salt Lake City, Utah, has used computerized systems to improve patient care for more than 25 years. In 1998, an article in the *New England Journal of Medicine* described the evaluation of LDS Hospital's computer-assisted management program for antibiotics and other antiinfective agents (Evans et al. 1998). (For more information on the details of the technology, see the reference list at the end of this chapter.) Managers must understand how the LDS Hospital's team defined the purpose of clinical information systems: "The project was designed to augment physicians' judgment, not to replace it. The computer was simply a tool that offered data on individual patients, decision logic, and prescribing information to physicians in a useful and non-threatening way" (Garibaldi 1998).

The purpose of the clinical information system was to support decision making, and this in turn fostered cooperation between informaticists and clinicians. Too often the purposes of a clinical information system are to control behavior rather than to support it, to reduce practitioner autonomy rather than enhance it, and to fulfill administrator requirements rather than fulfill patient and clinician requirements. These purposes foster adversarial rather than cooperative relationships. A clear description of the purpose can create common ground for the team and practitioners, contribute to their ability to focus on a common goal, and enlist practitioner buy-in to successfully use innovative technology to improve patient outcomes.

Promoting Breakthrough Ideas and Solutions

In Chapter 3, the process tool called "lead-time analysis" was introduced. The user of this tool physically walks through the steps of a process, notes the time it takes to complete a process step, measures the distance between steps, and analyzes the steps to determine if the process step contributes value to the overall process.

By using lead-time analysis, one team member of the laboratory redesign effort described earlier discovered the cumbersome and time-consuming process required for a test-result report to travel from the laboratory to the physician's office across the street. A clear understanding of the laboratory's purpose (to provide information) helped the team to ask the right questions before trying to improve this process. Previously the team might have asked, "How can we improve the process of delivering the results via the mail?" Instead, the team's understanding of purpose caused them to ask, "How can we get the information to the physician's office in the most timely manner?" By asking the improvement question this way, the team began to identify alternatives to mail and ultimately installed a fax server into the laboratory information system. The fax server enabled the laboratory to send test results directly to the fax machine in a physician's office to improve the timeliness with which customers received laboratory results while at the same time improving customer satisfaction (Kelly 1998).

This example may sound very basic; however, it also demonstrates the value of understanding purpose. Had the laboratory designed an intervention on the basis of its original purpose, the department might have improved the mail process or added staff to the customer service team. Instead, when it focused on its real purpose, the department was able to design a much more effective solution.

The Purpose Principle

The examples in this chapter illustrate that, as healthcare systems grow in complexity, it becomes easy to forget to periodically evaluate an organization's purpose. Managers must develop the habit of asking themselves, "What are we really trying to achieve? On the basis of changes in the environment, technology, or customer requirements, what is our purpose? Does our current method of operating serve that purpose, or are there more effective alternatives?" When the purpose is clear, new solutions usually become clear as well.

The purpose principle comes from the concept of breakthrough thinking (Nadler and Hibino 1994), an approach to problem solving developed from studying effective leaders and problem solvers from various industries and disciplines. Nadler and Hibino (1994, 1) found that "when confronted with a problem, successful people tend to question why they should spend their time and effort solving the problem at all" and that effective problem solvers "always placed every problem into a larger context...to understand the relationship between what effective action on the problem was supposed to achieve and the purposes of the larger setting of which the original problem was a part." By questioning purpose and enlarging the boundaries from which they examined the problem, effective problem solvers were able to purposely and systematically choose the right problem and, in turn, the best solution.

When examined from a systems thinking perspective, using the purpose principle promotes double-loop learning by challenging assumptions about the nature of a problem. By encouraging the viewing of the problem and solution from the larger context of the entire system, the purpose principle also promotes an understanding of the connections between the problem at hand and other elements or components of the system.

From Concept to Practice

A series of questions can help managers to examine and clarify purpose. The first question should be, "What am I trying to accomplish," or "What is this process, intervention, or department designed to accomplish?" By asking this question first, a discussion of purpose and accompanying mental models regarding the problem and solution may be brought into the open.

The next question involves expanding the purpose. Expanding the purpose is not meant to reduce the problem to a lesser problem but instead to identify and understand how the problem is related to the overall context in which it exists. Think of an onion. The effort of expanding the purpose is actually like starting from the inside of an onion and adding on the layers to construct a whole onion rather than peeling the onion, which is typically how the onion metaphor is used. When purpose is identified, questions like, "Why do we do that?" follow. In this way, the larger purposes may be identified—and more layers are added to the onion. When the original purpose has been expanded several times, then another question should be asked: "What larger purpose might eliminate the need to achieve this smaller purpose?" (Nadler and Hibino 1994, 154). Primary prevention approaches often provide solutions in this way. Rather than finding better ways to treat diseases caused by waterborne organisms, early public health practitioners devised ways to eliminate the organisms from drinking water. Similarly, vaccinations, like the polio vaccine, are solutions to a larger purpose (preventing the disease) rather than a smaller purpose (treating the disease).

By questioning, identifying, and documenting different purposes, the manager or team may then select the level of purpose most appropriate to solve, which is the purpose that enables them to solve the right problem and that is within their means (e.g., resources, scope of authority). At first the questions may be difficult to answer and may appear to be redundant. However, like anything new, with practice the ability to answer the questions will improve, and the repetition will encourage a deeper level of thinking about the problem.

Example One

Here is an example of how one might approach a problem using the purpose principle and might answer the aforementioned questions. A manager at a local community center is faced with the problem of inconsistent collection of fees for wellness classes sponsored by the center. Community center members have unlimited use of the swimming pool and exercise equipment. The center also offers members a variety of wellness classes for a small fee, which is intended to cover the cost of the instructors and materials. Some classes are taught at the center by the center's staff, but some are taught by instructors employed by local healthcare providers. For example, a class on low-fat menus may be sponsored by the wellness program but taught at the local hospital by the hospital's dietitian. Collecting fees for the classes offered on-site is not a problem because class participants are required to check in at the reception desk. However, for off-site classes the collection rate is barely 50 percent. The center has also received numerous complaints from course instructors that either too many or not enough participants showed up for a particular class.

The manager may ask herself the following questions (possible answers are in italics):

- What am I trying to accomplish?
  To collect fees from class enrollees.

- Have I expanded the purposes of addressing the problem? Why do I try to collect fees from class enrollees?
  To increase revenue we need to have accurate record keeping, including who has registered, who has attended, and who has paid for the class. We also have to make sure the fees we charge cover the costs of the class, instructors, and materials.

- What is the purpose of increasing revenues, having accurate record keeping, and covering the costs of instructors and material?
  To cover our own expenses if we want to continue to offer a wide variety of classes taught by quality instructors.

- What is the purpose of covering our expenses?
  To remain financially sound and to continue to provide wellness services for the community.

- What are my customers' purposes?
  The purposes of the instructors are to offer their classes with minimal logistics and administrative hassles (e.g., compensation, paperwork) and to be prepared for their classes. The purposes of the members are to stay healthy and to have a place for social interaction.

- What larger purpose may eliminate the need to achieve this smaller purpose altogether?
  If I had a grant or if community partners donated money, time, or staff, we would not have to worry about charging members and collecting fees.

- What is the right problem for me to be working on?
  To improve the logistics and administrative processes and to provide a low-hassle teaching environment for our instructors and low-hassle classes for our members.

Although the initial focus for this manager was to collect more money, after answering this series of questions, she realized that the center had not explicitly defined or communicated the roles and expectations of the community center staff, the class participants, or the class instructors for an off-site offering. One expectation was about how and when payment should be collected. As a result, the manager changed her focus from collecting money to defining and communicating expectations. She then identified a variety of interventions to help with this new purpose, including changing the content of class brochures and posters, holding an orientation meeting with off-site instructors, setting registration deadlines so a final participant roster could be faxed to instructors at least 24 hours in advance, and assigning a community-center staff member as a liaison to assist the instructor with logistics and fee collection. The manager also began to think about how she could engage financial support from local providers to help defray some of the costs.

Example Two

To further illustrate the purpose principle, here is another example of how it might be used. The administrator for a large multispecialty, ambulatory medical practice has implemented a new performance management system for the entire organization. When the office manager for one of the obstetrics and gynecology practices is given the first "clinic report card," the data show that, for obstetrics patients, the practice has performed very well in the area of pregnancy-associated complications. However, the practice has performed poorly in the areas of patient satisfaction. In particular, patients are not satisfied with their level of involvement in their own care and their preparation for labor, delivery, breast-feeding, and care of their newborns.

The manager knows staff members are committed to quality patient care and are very hard workers. Out of curiosity, the manager asks one of the obstetricians, "What is the purpose of prenatal care and the prenatal office visits?" The physician replies, "To identify signs of problems with the mother or the fetus and to intervene early to prevent problems from getting worse." The manager then asks the physician what kinds of problems could potentially occur, to which he replies, "Conditions like toxemia in the mother or growth retardation in the fetus."

The manager initially identifies the problem as patient dissatisfaction with prenatal care; the process to be improved as prenatal care; and, the purpose of the prenatal visits as described by the physician: early identification and intervention of problems with the mother and the fetus or baby. The manager then asks a series of purpose questions:

- What am I trying to accomplish?
  To improve the clinic's "report card" results in the area of patient dissatisfaction with prenatal care.

- Have I expanded the purposes of addressing this problem? What is the purpose of the clinic's "report card"?
  To monitor patient satisfaction with the care they receive in our clinic.

- Have I further expanded the purpose? What is the purpose of monitoring patient satisfaction with the care they receive in our clinic?
  To keep existing patients and to attract new patients to our clinic.

- Have I further expanded the purpose? What is the purpose of keeping existing patients and attracting new patients to our clinic?
  To stay in business and pay the bills.

- For physicians, what is the purpose of prenatal care?
  To identify signs of problems with the mother or the fetus and to intervene early to prevent problems from getting worse.

- For patients, what is the purpose of prenatal care?
  To have a healthy pregnancy and a healthy baby. To learn about prenatal classes and other parenting resources.

- For the insurance companies, what is the purpose of prenatal care?
  To prevent complications that require extended hospitalization of the mother or the baby and to keep overall healthcare costs down.

- What larger purpose would eliminate the need to achieve this smaller purpose altogether?
  If nobody got pregnant or had babies.

- What is the right purpose for me to be working on? How does this purpose differ or not differ from my original purpose?
  By answering these questions, it becomes apparent that the physicians, the office manager, the patients, and the insurance companies have somewhat different yet somewhat overlapping purposes. The purpose principle may be used to align all of these parties around a common purpose. A more comprehensive purpose for prenatal care that addresses all of the stakeholder requirements/purposes here would be more effective.

  For example: The purpose of the clinic's prenatal services is to assess, monitor, and manage the physiological and psychosocial needs of families during the childbearing process.

Once the purpose is defined, the activities to achieve that purpose may then be segmented according to the different stakeholders. It is often helpful to define the following corollaries to the purpose to ensure that the various stakeholders or discussion participants can see that their ideas are addressed. Examples of such corollaries include the following:

- The desired *results* are healthy clinical outcomes, satisfied patients, and cost-effective services.
- The clinic will *measure* how successful it is in achieving the desired

results with the following data: maternal and infant complication rates, early diagnosis, patient satisfaction, payer satisfaction, and so on.

- The *service mix, processes, and interventions* used to accomplish the purpose may then be strategically determined, designed and/or improved.

- The *goals* for performance improvement efforts may be to validate the purposes of the key stakeholders identified earlier; refine the clinic's purpose for prenatal care services based on any new information obtained; evaluate current practices to determine the extent to which the clinic is accomplishing its purpose; define a service mix that is consistent with the purpose; prioritize those services needing improvement; and design, redesign, and implement improved processes that meet all stakeholder requirements and accomplish our new definition of purpose. (This is a multiple, positive, clear goal incorporating partial or intermediate goals.)

Although the results of this example may seem intuitive or obvious, without the discussion of purpose, it is likely that the clinic manager would have set goals to improve the aesthetics surrounding care, rather than the actual care processes themselves, to improve patient satisfaction.

Conclusion

This chapter introduces the concept and role of purpose in quality management. The companion readings section below lists works that provide a detailed description of the purpose principle and an in-depth explanation of how managers may approach it. The exercise at the end of this chapter has been designed to provide an opportunity for readers to practice the purpose principle and become more acquainted with how to apply this concept to a healthcare problem. Chapter 10 discusses the role of measurement in quality management and offers measurement lessons from a systems thinking perspective.

Companion Readings

Nadler, G., and S. Hibino. 1994. *Breakthrough Thinking: The Seven Principles of Creative Problem Solving*, 17–37, 127–59. Rocklin, CA: Prima Publishing.

Repenning, N. P., and J. D. Sterman. 2001. "Nobody Ever Gets Credit for Fixing Problems That Never Happened: Creating and Sustaining Process Improvement." *California Management Review* 43 (4): 64–88.

References

Evans, R. S., S. L. Pestotnik, D. C. Classen, T. P. Clemmer, L. K. Weaver, J. F. Orme, J. F. Lloyd, and J. P. Burke. 1998. "A Computer-Assisted

Management Program for Antibiotics and Other Antiinfective Agents." *New England Journal of Medicine* 338 (4): 232–38.

Garibaldi, R. A. 1998. "Computers and the Quality of Care—A Clinician's Perspective." *New England Journal of Medicine* 338 (4): 259–60.

Jencks, S. F., E. D. Huff, and T. Cuerdon. 2003. "Change in the Quality of Care Delivered to Medicare Beneficiaries, 1998–1999 to 2000–2001." *JAMA* 289 (3): 305–12.

Jha, A. K., Z. Li, E. J. Orav, and A. M. Epstein. 2005. "Care in U.S. Hospitals—The Hospital Quality Alliance Program." *New England Journal of Medicine* 353 (3): 265–74.

Kelly, D. L. 1998. "Reframing Beliefs About Work and Change Processes in Redesigning Laboratory Services." *Joint Commission Journal on Quality Improvement* 24 (9): 154–67.

Kelly, D. L., S. L. Pestotnik, M. C. Coons, and J. W. Lelis. 1997. "Reengineering a Surgical Service Line: Focusing on Core Process Improvement." *American Journal of Medical Quality* 12 (2): 120–29.

Nadler, G., and S. Hibino. 1994. *Breakthrough Thinking: The Seven Principles of Creative Problem Solving*. Rocklin, CA: Prima Publishing.

Exercise

Objectives: To practice using the purpose principle and to better understand how purpose and goals are linked.

Instructions

1. This exercise builds on the topic of the Hospital Quality Alliance, introduced in the Chapter 8 exercise. The study results are shown again below.

    Analysis of data from the [Hospital Quality Alliance] national reporting system shows that performance varies among hospitals and across indicators.... [P]erformance scores for acute myocardial infarction closely predicted performance scores for congestive health failure but not for pneumonia.... [O]ur findings indicate that quality measures had only moderate predictive ability across the three conditions. Although a high quality of care for acute myocardial infarction predicted a high quality of care for congestive heart failure, the former was only marginally better than chance for identifying a high quality of care for pneumonia. These data do not provide support for the notion that 'good' hospitals are easy to identify or consistent in their performance across conditions (Jha et al. 2005, 265, 272).

2. Read the following scenario.

> You are the CEO of a large, tertiary care hospital. You have closely followed your own hospital's performance on the Hospital Quality Alliance Performance Indicators, which have shown minor, yet steady, improvement over the past year. When the Hospital Compare website went live, for the first time you were able to analyze and compare your organization's performance with that of the other hospitals in your community, in your state, and across the nation. Your percentile rankings are disappointing. As with other hospital boards of directors, your board has been taking a more active interest and role in quality of care. You want to propose performance improvement goals along with the Hospital Compare results at the next board meeting; however, the medical director for the cardiac service line just showed you the *New England Journal of Medicine* article quoted above. The article brings to mind a question someone asked you several months ago: teaching smoking cessation is a requirement for congestive heart failure, AMI, and pneumonia. Why does the hospital have three different processes to address smoking cessation and three different results in the CMS indicator to comply with teaching smoking cessation, depending on the disease?

3. Practice the purpose principle by writing your responses to the following questions:
   a. What am I trying to accomplish?
   b. Have I expanded the purposes of addressing this problem? What is the purpose of the process or activities involved in response to a?
   c. Have I further expanded the purpose? What is the purpose of response to b?
   d. Have I further expanded the purpose? What is the purpose of response to c?
   e. Have I further expanded the purpose? What is the purpose of response to d?
   f. For the patients, what is the purpose?
   g. For clinical staff, what is the purpose?
   h. What larger purpose may eliminate the need to achieve this smaller purpose altogether?
   i. What is the right purpose for me to be working on? Describe how this purpose differs or does not differ from my original purpose.
   j. Review your responses to the questions above. Given your understanding of purpose, what goals will you present to your board of directors?

4. Compare the goals you selected in #3.j to the goal you selected in Chapter 7 exercise #5. Describe how they are similar or different.

PERFORMANCE MEASUREMENT

Objectives

- To describe the essential role of measurement in quality management
- To present systems lessons on using performance measurement
- To introduce concepts related to process variation
- To explore sources of comparative data

Baseball scores, the weather report, interest rates, and even grass height satisfy our need for measurement. We are accustomed to using data to make decisions and monitor our personal interests, whether we are following the progress of our favorite sports team, determining how to dress, deciding to buy a house, or knowing when to mow the lawn.

People use data to guide their own healthcare activities, too. A child's hot forehead alerts a mother to the possibility of a fever. A grandfather with diabetes measures his daily blood glucose level to regulate his insulin dosage. People exercise 20 minutes a day, three times a week to remain fit. Care providers use data to diagnose, treat, and monitor clinical conditions and the effectiveness of interventions. Blood tests, x-rays, and vital signs all provide information to enhance the care provider's effectiveness. In each of these examples, data add value to the process. Data give us information about something we are interested in, help us to choose among various options, alert us when something needs to be done, and define the boundaries of an activity.

When we follow our favorite sports team during the course of the season, we are looking at data over time for trends and progress. When we check to see what place the team is in relation to the other teams in the same division, we are comparing data points. When we realize the grass is high compared with the neighbors', we are using a benchmark to signal that we need to mow it. If we check the weather report for the barometric pressure or chance of rain, we are using formal measures. When we use our hand to check a forehead for fever, we are measuring informally.

Healthcare managers often forget these measurement lessons from other parts of life. In healthcare organizations, measurement may occur by default—that is, we measure what we can measure. Measurement may occur because it is required by regulatory agencies such as JCAHO, and rules from other industries may dictate measurement systems such as monthly, quarterly, or annual financial statements. While immersed in data and reporting, healthcare managers face the risk of being "data rich and information poor" about how their unit, department, or organization is actually performing.

This chapter discusses measurement as the foundation for organizational effectiveness, lists several systems lessons for using measurement in improving and managing performance, and reviews process variation that affects quality.

The Foundation for Organizational Effectiveness

Although a manager may successfully report the performance indicators required by internal and external stakeholders, she may still not be successfully managing her organization. Managers must recognize the difference between reporting indicators and measuring performance. According to the Baldrige National Quality Program Healthcare Criteria (NIST 2006, 6), "measurement, analysis and knowledge-management are critical to the effective management of your organization and to a fact-based, knowledge-driven system for improving health care and operational performance" and "serve as a foundation for the performance management system." In other words, measurement is essential to managing and improving organizational performance and results. Therefore, managers must see performance—not simply performance indicators—as the end result of their efforts.

The thought of designing, implementing, and using performance measures may seem overwhelming at first to a healthcare manager. However, when performance measurement is viewed as a process, steps may be taken to initiate, carry out, and continually improve the process. Figure 10.1 describes a continuum that a manager or organization may use to determine the maturity of a performance measurement system. As shown in Figure 10.1, those embarking on new or early efforts are on the far left of the continuum and may have few or no reported results. Those who are experienced in their efforts are shown on the far right and are characterized by not only what and how performance is reported but also by results that demonstrate improvement over time and show leadership within their industries (NIST 2006).

In recent years, availability of and access to comparative data in healthcare have greatly improved. The web resources at the end of the chapter provide data sources that managers may use in comparing their organizations' performance to that of other organizations.

Lessons for Healthcare Managers

Managers must purposefully select indicators and design a measurement system that is linked to and aligned with their organizations' goals, business

FIGURE 10.1

The Continuum of Maturity in Performance Measurement

There are no results or poor results in areas reported

There are some improvements and/or early good performance levels in a few areas

Results are not reported for many to most areas of importance to your key organizational requirements

Improvements and/or good performance levels are reported in many areas of importance to your key organizational requirements

Early stages of developing trends and obtaining comparative information are evident

Results are reported for many to most areas of importance to your key organizational requirements

Improvement trends and/or good performance levels are reported for most areas of importance to your key organizational requirements

No pattern of adverse trends and no poor performance levels are evident in areas of importance to your key organizational requirements

Some trends and/or current performance levels—evaluated against relevant comparisons and/or benchmarks—show areas of strength and/or good to very good relative performance levels

Organizational performance results address most key customer, market, and process requirements

Beginning Efforts ⟶ **Mature Efforts**

Source: Adapted from National Institute of Standards and Technology. 2006. "Baldrige National Quality Program Health Care Criteria for Performance Excellence." Gaithersburg, MD: National Institute of Standards and Technology.

strategy, and customer and stakeholder requirements. Managers should also consider the lessons in this section when selecting and using indicators in a performance measurement system.

Choose a Balanced Set of Measures

Managers should use a varied and balanced set of measures or indicators to ensure that one area of performance is not unintentionally excelling at the expense of another.

An approach called the balanced scorecard has been described in business literature (Kaplan and Norton 1992, 1993, 1996; *Harvard Management Update* 2000) and in healthcare literature (Aidemark 2001; Chow et al. 1998; Inamdar, Kaplan, and Bower 2002; Inamdar et al. 2000; Jason 2001; Zelman et al. 1999). The balanced scorecard is a "set of measures that gives top managers a fast but comprehensive view of the business" (Kaplan and Norton 1992, 71). Data are reported in specific categories that represent four perspectives of the organization's performance: (1) the customer perspective, (2) the internal perspective, (3) the innovation and learning perspective, and (4) the financial perspective (Kaplan and Norton 1992).

The clinical value compass may be thought of as a balanced scorecard for evaluating outcomes of a clinical process. The four categories that it measures (the points of the compass) are functional status and well-being, satisfaction against need, costs, and clinical status (Nelson et al. 1996). These four points may be used to measure, evaluate, and improve the effectiveness of a clinical process, and they may also serve as a guide for managers when selecting metrics to measure, evaluate, and improve the performance of their departments or organizations (Kelly et al. 1997).

When choosing performance indicators, managers must balance the categories (e.g., using the balanced scorecard or using clinical value compass approaches) and the types of measures. The three types of medical quality indicators are structure measures, process measures, and outcome measures. Tools, resources, characteristics of providers, settings, and organizations are considered structure measures (Donabedian 1980); examples of these types of measures are the number of hospital beds, the number of physicians on staff, and the age of the radiology equipment. Activities that occur between patients and providers—in other words, what is done to the patient—are considered process measures (Brook, Kamberg, and McGlynn 1996; Fitzgerald, Moore, and Dittus 1988). Preventive care activities, such as mammography, immunization, and prenatal care during the first trimester, are examples of process measures. Many of the CMS indicators discussed in chapters 8 and 9 are also examples of process measures. Changes in clinical status—in other words, what happens to the patient—are considered outcome measures (Brook, Kamberg, and McGlynn 1996; Donabedian 1980). The number of enrolled women who get a mammogram is a process measure, while the number of women who die from breast cancer is an outcome measure.

These three types of measures should also be considered when defining and selecting operational and management indicators. The proportion of new graduates to experienced staff is a structure measure, the number of staff who attended an in-service education class is a process measure, and the number of patient complaints is an outcome measure.

Translate Data into Information

Measures should reflect the performance of the entity that is being managed; therefore, a large hospital may have several levels and scopes of measurement. The CEO may review hospitalwide measures, a service line manager may focus on measures for a specific group of departments or patients, a department manager may focus on measures for that department, and a shift supervisor may focus on measures for a particular shift. All levels of performance indicators should reflect the common direction and priorities defined by the organization's mission, vision, and business strategy. A comprehensive performance measurement system should also ensure coordination among levels to minimize the duplication of collecting, reporting, and analyzing efforts.

Note that, as data are aggregated, some performance information may become buried in the data and that important opportunities for evaluation and improvement may be missed. For example, throughout the 1990s, hospital administrators used a common strategy of changing the ratio of professional staff and assistant personnel to reduce the average hourly wage expenses and in turn the overall personnel costs. Administrators of a large tertiary care hospital that used this staffing strategy tracked staff turnover rates as one of the hospital's performance indicators. In 1995, turnover for the nursing department was at 25 percent, which the administrators considered to be reasonable given the local employment and economic environments. However, the nurse managers and nurses consistently voiced their concerns about understaffing and turnover.

When different levels of the organization are telling different stories about the operating environment, unbundling or disaggregating the indicators can be a useful strategy to evaluate the appropriateness of performance measures. When the nursing department's turnover data were examined more closely, all personnel in the department were found to be included in the calculations of turnover. The aggregate turnover figures reflected the combined turnover of registered nurses, licensed practical nurses, certified nurse assistants, and unit secretaries. Although the departmental turnover was 25 percent, the registered nurse turnover was 15 percent and the certified nursing assistant turnover was 43 percent. The potential salary savings for the lower-paid certified nursing assistants were essentially neutralized by the cost of recruiting, hiring, and training the constantly changing stream of these assistants.

In addition, while studying the departmental turnover data, the human resources department realized that internal staff transfers were not included in the turnover calculations; only terminations were included. When staff movement within the organization was also taken into account, the turnover figures significantly underestimated the impact of staff changes on both the nursing managers and the frontline nursing staffs. Once these flaws in the performance indicators were identified, the human resources department redesigned its performance indicators and reporting mechanisms to account for changing activity at the unit level in addition to aggregate turnover at the departmental or organizational level.

Evaluate Specific Interventions and Ongoing Performance

A manager may evaluate both the performance of a specific intervention and ongoing performance. The Shewhart cycle (see Chapter 3) provides a framework for collecting and reviewing data for a specific improvement intervention. This type of evaluation is illustrated by an improvement effort conducted by a group of anesthesiologists. When a new protocol for preoperative laboratory test requirements was implemented, the follow-up measurement was important to evaluate both the degree to which the protocol was being followed and the impact of the new protocol on test use. One year later, evaluation data showed that unnecessary blood tests performed on patients undergoing tonsillectomy/adenoidectomy surgery declined by 51 percent and that unnecessary blood tests on patients undergoing arthroscopic knee surgery declined by 38 percent (Kelly et al. 1997).

For ongoing operations, the Shewhart cycle suggests that managers should review performance indicators on a regular basis; plan appropriate interventions, if needed; implement appropriate solutions; and then continue to review performance indicators regularly. Some indicators, such as patient census, may be reported daily, weekly, monthly, quarterly, and annually. The reporting interval for a specific indicator will depend on customer and stakeholder requirements, intended uses, and organizational capabilities and resources. For example, measures used for ongoing operations in a multisite surgical services division included patient volumes, cost, patient satisfaction, clinical outcomes, and indicators related to specific service-line improvement goals for that year. At monthly manager meetings, in addition to a more detailed monthly financial report, each manager received two performance reports: a service-line performance report and a site-specific performance report. During these meetings, the managers reviewed, analyzed, and discussed the data; identified both good performance trends and areas of concern; and explored potential solutions and interventions. The check/study, act, and plan stages of the Shewhart cycle took place in a collaborative fashion among the unit managers in the service line. In the time between the monthly meetings, the managers were responsible for the "do" stage of the cycle, if required. By doing this, the management team used a monthly Shewhart cycle to incorporate the performance measures into the overall performance management system (Kelly et al. 1997).

Understand the Relationship Between System and Component Measures

Historically, functional management structures in healthcare organizations have promoted component measures. It is not uncommon for hospitals to measure department-specific costs per unit of service. The laboratory may measure costs per test, while the pharmacy may measure costs per prescription. Because patients receive care from multiple departments within the hospital or along the continuum of care, managers must recognize and balance component and system costs from the organization's point of view and the patient's point of view.

For example, from the organization's point of view, the cost of an expensive drug from the pharmacy is acceptable if the drug allows the patient's overall length of stay to be reduced. Alternatively, the hospital can reduce the cost of an episode of care by cutting its discharge planner positions and thereby reducing its personnel expense. From the patient's point of view, however, an unnecessary readmission to the hospital can be avoided if the patient receives adequate home care instructions from a discharge planner. Although the hospital may be able to save money on a single episode of care, the overall cost of care to the healthcare system will increase because of a readmission that could have been avoided if adequate discharge preparation had been offered the first time.

Managers, especially at higher levels in the organization, must be conscious of the interrelationships between system and component measures as they are establishing departmental and organizational performance direction and goals. When measures are viewed from a systems perspective, some components of the system may be intentionally suboptimized to optimize performance of the entire system. Likewise, some components of the system may be unintentionally optimized at the expense of the performance of the entire system.

Consider the redesign of an ambulatory surgery unit as an example. The redesign revealed that, as the clinical protocol for preoperative laboratory tests was revised to eliminate unnecessary tests (Kelly et al. 1997), the remaining blood tests could be conducted using point-of-care testing instruments. This new process eliminated the need for specimens to be transported to the hospital laboratory to be analyzed and for the results to be communicated back to the unit. The streamlined process cut 30 to 45 minutes from the preoperative length of stay. If the decision to go with the point-of-care testing had been made solely on the basis of cost per test, the new process would not have been implemented; the point-of-care cost per test was about five times greater than when the procedure was done in the laboratory. However, the savings and efficiencies gained by reducing unnecessary preoperative length of stay far outweighed the few dollars of difference in the cost per laboratory test.

Balancing system and component measures when allocating departmental resources and monitoring the impact of improvement efforts require collaboration, negotiation, and awareness of the larger picture. The example in Chapter 9 concerning the laboratory's purpose also shows the need for negotiation and intentionally addressing the issue of system and component measures. The hospital in which the laboratory operated used the practice of benchmarking to establish performance targets for its managers. This laboratory demonstrated a higher cost per test than the benchmark data. The definition of purpose, however, enabled the manager to describe to the administrator that, although the higher cost per test reflected the expense incurred by the laboratory for consulting with other units, the benefit of savings was realized by other units or the hospital overall. The administrator and manager could then set more appropriate performance targets that take into account the differences between the practice of this laboratory and the practices that generated the benchmarking data.

Balancing system and component measures becomes more of a challenge when addressing continuum-of-care issues. Managers may include measures of unintended consequences in their overall performance measures to better understand the impact of their own interventions on others. In Chapter 4, an example is introduced that illustrates dynamic complexity in healthcare systems. Look at this same example from a measurement perspective. Following is a review of the example. The advent of prospective payment systems in the 1980s drove many hospitals to cut costs by reducing length of stay. An unintended consequence of this practice was that it shifted the monetary, functional, and quality-of-life costs to a downstream service or unit in the continuum of care or to the patients themselves. Table 4.1 illustrates the unintended consequences of reducing hospital length of stay for patients who received total hip arthroplasty.

Managers, financial officers, CEOs, and policymakers must all be aware of how decisions made and implemented within their domains of responsibility affect other parts of the healthcare system, both positively and negatively. They should ask themselves the following questions:

- Who is affected by this intervention?
- Who affects this intervention?
- What are possible unintended consequences of this intervention?
- Am I measuring the right thing?
- Have I included a measure of unintended consequences in my evaluation of the intervention?
- Am I unintentionally shifting costs to another component of the healthcare system?

Integrate Stakeholder Requirements

Chapters 2 and 6 discuss the increasing role of external stakeholders in establishing quality requirements. When managers are considering and selecting a balanced set of measures, they should take into account these stakeholder requirements. Managers may categorize clinical and satisfaction measures (clinical value compass) or customer measures (balanced scorecard) into the following categories set forth by the Institute of Medicine (2001, 7) in "Envisioning the National Health Care Quality Report":

- Safety refers to avoiding injuries to patients from care that is intended to help them.
- Effectiveness refers to providing services based on scientific knowledge to all who could benefit and refraining from providing services to those not likely to benefit (avoiding overuse and misuse).
- Patient centeredness refers to healthcare that establishes a partnership among practitioners, patients, and their families (when appropriate) to ensure that decisions respect patients' wants, needs, and preferences and that patients have the education and support they require to make decisions and participate in their own care.
- Timeliness refers to obtaining needed care and minimizing unnecessary delays in getting that care.

The report goes on to suggest the additional categories from the consumer's perspective of staying healthy, getting better, living with an illness or disability, and coping with the end of life (IOM 2001, 7). These categories provide the framework for the Agency for Healthcare Research and Quality's National Healthcare Quality Report.

Figure 10.1 offers a maturity continuum to guide managers in designing, implementing, and using performance measures to manage the organization. When the role of reporting requirements for external stakeholders is added to the equation, managers are compelled to move along the quality continuum described in Chapter 1. Figure 10.2 further enhances an understanding of the quality continuum by describing the continuum for organizational effectiveness. To move along this continuum, managers must not only measure performance relative to internal operations and local requirements but must also align and integrate measurement approaches with requirements of stakeholders of the larger healthcare system.

Integrating internal and external measurement requirements may also be thought of in terms of a Venn diagram. In Figure 10.3, one circle represents internally driven performance measures, while the other circle represents externally driven performance measures. To leverage time, effort, and resources, managers should strategically select measures that allow for the largest area of overlap between the circles. In this way, performance measures may be used for multiple purposes both internally and externally.

Process Variation

Anyone who depends on public transportation has firsthand experience with process variation. If you have missed a bus because the driver was

FIGURE 10.2

Organizational Effectiveness Continuum for Healthcare Managers

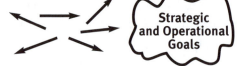

(1) Reacting to Problems

Strategic and Operational Goals

Operations are characterized by activities rather than by processes, and they are largely responsive to immediate needs or problems. Goals are poorly defined.

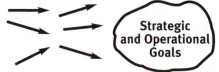

(2) Early Systematic Approaches

Strategic and Operational Goals

The organization is at the beginning stages of conducting operations by processes with repeatability, evaluation and improvement, and some early coordination among organizational units. Strategy and quantitative goals are being defined.

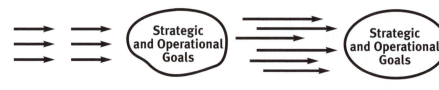

(3) Aligned Approaches

Strategic and Operational Goals

Operations are characterized by processes that are repeatable and regularly evaluated for improvement, with learnings shared and with coordination among organizational units. Processes address key strategies and goals of the organization.

(4) Integrated Approaches

Strategic and Operational Goals

Operations are characterized by processes that are repeatable and regularly evaluated for change and improvement in collaboration with other affected units. Efficiencies across units are sought and achieved through analysis, innovation, and sharing. Processes and measures track progress on key strategic and operational goals.

Source: National Institute of Standards and Technology. 2006. "Baldrige National Quality Program Healthcare Criteria for Performance Excellence," 56. Gaithersburg, MD: National Institute of Standards and Technology.

ahead of schedule or if you have been late for work because the driver was behind schedule, you have experienced the inconvenience and cost of variation in a process.

In Chapter 1, the goals of quality improvement are described as improving average performance and reducing the unnecessary variation from the average to ensure more consistent results each time the process is carried out. These goals are illustrated with a frequency distribution in Figure 1.3. A statistical process control chart is a valuable tool that can help managers monitor, identify, explain, and manage variation in performance data. An in-depth explanation of statistical process control charts is beyond the scope of this

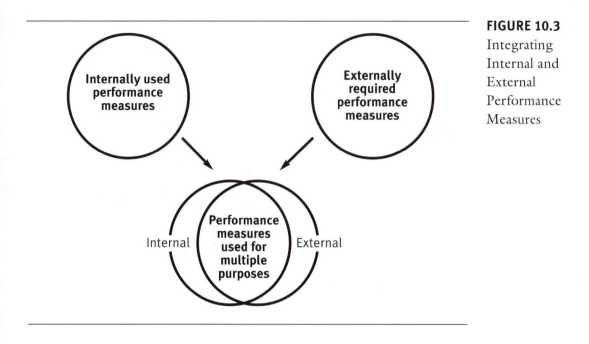

FIGURE 10.3
Integrating
Internal and
External
Performance
Measures

book. However, in this section an overview of the basic concepts is presented to help a manager understand and use statistical process control charts.

Statistical Process Control Charts

A statistical process control chart is a way of displaying performance data to enhance a manager's ability to identify variation in performance. Think of a process that is performed many times. The results are plotted on a frequency distribution, with the x-axis representing the value observed and the y-axis representing the number of times that value is observed. If the process is measured many times, a normal distribution—a bell curve—begins to take shape. Several measures may be derived from this normal distribution, including a measure of central tendency, such as a mean or average, and a measure of spread or distance from the mean, such as a standard deviation.

The total range of performance of the process is essentially captured by the values bounded by the mean plus three standard deviations above and below the mean. The boundaries established by the mean plus or minus two standard deviations will capture the process approximately 95 percent of the time (see Figure 10.4). When the frequency distribution is turned on its side, with the x-axis showing increments of time (e.g., day, month, quarter) and the y-axis showing the performance for that time period, the manager has constructed a control chart (see Figure 10.5). In this way, the manager may track and compare performance over time.

A manager may get started using control charts with a few underlying concepts. First, "the Voice of the Customer defines what you want from a system" (Wheeler 2000, 79). This phrase is another way of stating the

Key Concepts

FIGURE 10.4

Frequency
Distribution

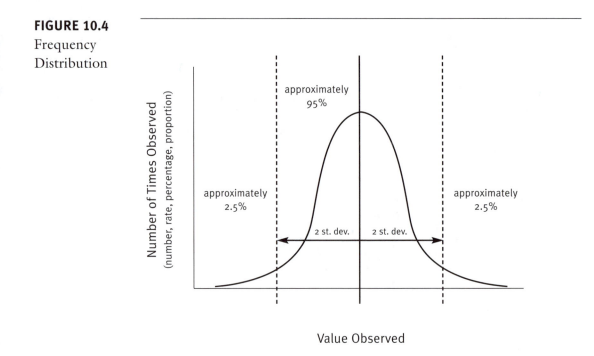

concepts of customer expectations and of patient and other stakeholder requirements that were introduced in Chapter 2. If an organization desires to be customer- or patient-focused, its processes must be rooted in the requirements of its patients, customers, and other stakeholders. The term "patient focused" does not mean simply being nice to patients or keeping them happy. Patient or customer focus means that the requirements of these groups are the foundation for and drive all work performed by the organization. In turn, organizational processes are designed with the intended result of meeting the requirements of patients, customers, and other stakeholders.

Second, "the Voice of the Process defines what you will get from a system" (Wheeler 2000, 79). This phrase defines the concept of process performance data. The work of the organization is accomplished through its processes, and the measure of the outcome or process output may be thought of as the "voice of the process." Just as the manager listens to the "voice of the customer" through such avenues as focus groups, satisfaction surveys, regulatory requirements, and reimbursement rates, the manager can listen to the "voice of the process" through control charts.

"It is management's job to work to bring the Voice of the Process into alignment with the Voice of the Customer.... If one is not pleased with the amount of variation shown by the Natural Process Limits, then one must go to work on the system, to change the underlying process rather than setting arbitrary goals, jawboning the workers, or looking for alternative ways of computing the limits" (Wheeler 2000, 44, 79). If process

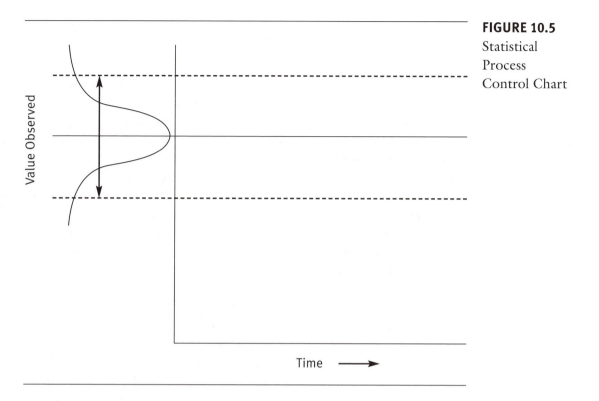

FIGURE 10.5

Statistical
Process
Control Chart

outputs show wide swings over time, the process was likely designed in such a manner that it delivers inconsistent rather than steady results. Adding training, working harder, or setting new goals will be ineffective strategies to improve the output of this process.

A manager must be able to recognize the two types of variation illustrated by control charts. *Random variation,* also referred to as noise or common cause variation, is the natural variation present in the process. *Assignable variation,* also referred to as a signal, indicates that a change in the process has occurred. The manager can distinguish random variation as those points that lie within the boundaries of the upper and lower control limits. Assignable or special cause variation is present when the manager sees any of the following situations (Wheeler 2000):

- A value that is above the upper control limit or below the lower control limit
- Three to four successive values that lie closer to the control limits than to the mean
- Eight or more consecutive points that lie on the same side of the mean

The reason that a manager must be able to distinguish between random and assignable variation is that she will need to respond differently, depending on the type of variation present. A manager cannot do anything to change the amount of random variation exhibited by the process except to change, redesign, or improve the underlying process itself. Assignable variation results from a distinct cause that may be investigated and identified by the manager. Once identified, the manager may eliminate or simply explain the cause.

Example

The following example illustrates how a manager may integrate statistical process control charts into hospital operations. In this example, the process being studied involves scheduling patient surgeries and allocating staff as needed. The voice of the customer includes the hospital administration, which requires cost-effective use of staffing dollars; physicians, who require the availability of a skilled operating room team; and employees, who require a satisfactory distribution of work hours. Figure 10.6 tracks the number of employee overtime hours for an operating room over four years.

In control charts, it is not uncommon to group data into time periods and to calculate the mean and control limits on the basis of the time periods selected. In this example, the end of the annual budget cycle is a natural cutoff point. As Figure 10.6 shows, each point indicates the actual number of overtime hours worked (y-axis) during each of the 26 pay periods in the calendar year (x-axis). The mean number of overtime hours for the year is shown as the center line, with the upper and lower control limits set at two standard deviations above and below the mean, respectively. In Year 1, Point A and Point B alert the manager to assignable variation. Upon investigation, the manager discovers that, during these two pay periods, in addition to staff absences because of vacation leaves, several staff had also attended professional conferences. Although the scheduling policy limited the number of staff who could be absent for vacation at one time and the number of staff who could be sent to workshops at one time, the policy failed to take into account the two instances of absences. By understanding this root cause, the manager redesigns the scheduling policy to limit the number of staff who could simultaneously be scheduled to be absent for any reason.

The portion of the control chart showing data for Year 2 provides the manager with another warning by showing increased variability in how the process is performing, which is indicated by the wider distance between the upper and lower control limits as well as by an increase in the average number of overtime hours per pay period. This pattern in the random variation indicates that the process did not perform as effectively as it had during the previous year. (Note that if the original mean and control limits were extended from Year 1 into Year 2, the consecutive values above the mean would alert the manager that something has changed in the process. In this case, patient volumes were increasing, but the scheduling process remained the same.) Point C alerts the manager to assignable variation. When the manager investigates the reason for this variation, she finds that it was caused by a large number of employees or their dependents being ill with the flu. The manager knows the cause, and the variation is expected to be a one-time occurrence, so it is simply explained.

In Year 3, the variability in the process continued to increase, and the situation was just about unmanageable. Growing patient volumes were

FIGURE 10.6
Control Chart Example

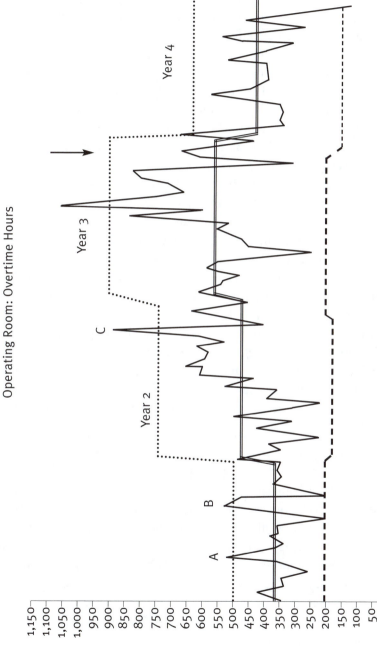

Operating Room: Overtime Hours

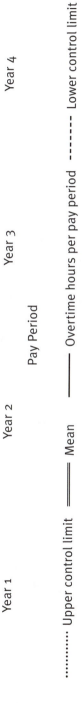

exacerbated by staff burnout and turnover. At that time, the manager knew that the scheduling process needed to be redesigned, so she asked a management engineer to analyze the situation and recommend solutions. The interventions (indicated by the arrow) included increasing the baseline number of staff to match the requirements of the growing patient volumes and redistributing staff across shifts to minimize peaks and valleys that had evolved over time to accommodate personnel preferences rather than patient needs.

The performance of the redesigned scheduling process is seen in the Year 4 pay periods. The change resulted in a decrease in the mean number of overtime hours by approximately 30 percent and a decrease in the variability (standard deviation) by about 30 percent. Although not yet as effective as the process in Year 1, the new scheduling process is a considerable improvement from the previous two years.

The intentions of this example are to illustrate the difference between random and assignable variations, to describe examples of interventions that a manager may use, and to illustrate that a control chart can show whether a management change can improve the performance of a process. In this example, the control chart was actually constructed retrospectively to better represent the impact of implementing the management engineer's recommendations. The negative results of the process had enough of an impact on both the manager and the employees to warrant the staffing analysis. Although the manager reviewed overtime hours pay period by pay period, she did not realize the extent to which the process had been out of control until the data were graphed in a control chart. Had the manager been adding the values to the chart as they occurred, the signals could have been observed and action could have been taken in a more timely way.

Conclusion

Performance measurement is essential to performance improvement. Although techniques for collecting, analyzing, and reporting data fall within the quantitative skill set of the organization, translating data into information that managers need to promote performance improvement requires a different and more subtle skill set. This chapter offers measurement examples, insights, and lessons for managers to help them better understand the performance of the systems in which they operate.

The exercise at the end of this chapter provides an opportunity to explore the "National Healthcare Quality Report." Chapter 11 describes concepts related to initiating and sustaining performance improvement.

Companion Readings

Kelly, D. L., and S. P. Johnson. 2005. "Measurement and Statistical Analysis in CQI." In *Continuous Quality Improvement in Health Care: Theory,*

Implementations, and Applications, 3rd edition., edited by C. P.
McLaughlin and A. D. Kaluzny, 95–109. Sudbury, MA: Jones and
Bartlett Publishers.

Wheeler, D. J. 2000. *Understanding Variation: The Key to Managing Chaos,
2nd edition*. Knoxville, TN: SPC Press.

Web Resources

Patient Satisfaction

NRC+Picker (National Research Corporation and the Picker Institute):
    nrcpicker.com
Press Ganey Associates: www.pressganey.com
The Gallup Organization: healthcare.gallup.com

Practice Patterns

Leatherman, S., and D. McCarthy. 2002. *Quality of Healthcare in the
    United States: A Chartbook*. New York: The Commonwealth Fund.
    www.cmwf.org/publications/publications_show.htm?doc_id=221238
The Center for the Evaluative Clinical Sciences, Dartmouth Medical School.
    1996. *The Dartmouth Atlas of Healthcare*. Chicago: The American
    Hospital Publishing Company. www.dartmouthatlas.org/

Health Plans

National Committee for Quality: www.ncqa.org

Clinical Indicators

Joint Commission on Accreditation of Healthcare Organizations
    Quality Check: www.qualitycheck.org
Centers for Medicare and Medicaid Services Medicare Clinical Indicators

- Hospital Compare (disease specific clinical indicators):
  www.hospitalcompare.hhs.gov

- Nursing Home Quality Initiative with link to Nursing Home Compare
  (long-term and short-stay indicators): www.cms.hhs.gov/quality/nhqi

- Home Health Quality Initiative with link to Home Health Compare
  (Home Health Outcome and Assessment Information Set or OASIS
  indicators): www.cms.hhs.gov/quality/hhqi

- Physician Focused Quality Initiative (Ambulatory Care):
  www.cms.hhs.gov/quality/pfqi.asp

Population Measures

State and local health departments
Centers for Disease Control and Prevention, National Center for
    Health Statistics: www.cdc.gov/nchs
The National Healthcare Quality Report: www.qualitytools.ahrq.gov
The National Healthcare Disparities Report: www.qualitytools.ahrq.gov

References

Aidemark, L. G. 2001. "The Meaning of Balanced Scorecard in the Healthcare Organisation." *Financial Accountability and Management* 17 (1): 23–40.

Brook, R. H., C. J. Kamberg, and E. McGlynn. 1996. "Health System Reform and Quality." *JAMA* 276 (6): 476–80.

Chow, C. W., D. Ganulin, O. Teknika, K. Haddad, and J. Williamson. 1998. "The Balanced Scorecard: A Potent Tool for Energizing and Focusing Healthcare Organization Management." *Journal of Healthcare Management* 43 (3): 263–80.

Donabedian, A. 1980. *Explorations in Quality Assessment and Monitoring, Volume I: The Definition of Quality and Approaches to Its Assessment.* Chicago: Health Administration Press.

Fitzgerald, J. F., P. S. Moore, and R. S. Dittus. 1988. "The Care of Elderly Patients with Hip Fracture. Changes Since Implementation of the Prospective Payment System." *New England Journal of Medicine* 319 (21): 1392–97.

Harvard Management Update. 2000. "The Balanced Scorecard's Lessons for Managers." *Harvard Management Update* 5 (10): 4–5.

Inamdar, N., R. S. Kaplan, and M. Bower. 2002. "Applying the Balanced Scorecard in Healthcare Provider Organizations." *Journal of Healthcare Management* 47 (3): 179–95.

Inamdar, N., R. S. Kaplan, M. L. Jones, and R. Menitoff. 2000. "The Balanced Scorecard: A Strategic Management System for Multi-Sector Collaboration and Strategy Implementation." *Quality Management in Healthcare* 8 (4): 21–39.

Institute of Medicine (IOM). 2001. *Envisioning the National Health Care Quality Report*, edited by M. H. Hurtado, E. K. Swift, and J. M. Corrigan. Washington, DC: National Academies Press.

Jason, O. 2001. "The Balanced Scorecard: An Integrative Approach to Performance Evaluation." *Healthcare Financial Management* 55 (5): 42–46.

Kaplan, R. S., and D. P. Norton. 1992. "The Balanced Scorecard—Measures that Drive Performance." *Harvard Business Review* 70 (1): 71–79.

———. 1993. "Putting the Balanced Scorecard to Work." *Harvard Business Review* 71 (5): 134–39.

———. 1996. *The Balanced Scorecard: Translating Strategy into Action.* Boston: Harvard Business School Press.

Kelly, D. L., S. L. Pestotnik, M. C. Coons, and J. W. Lelis. 1997. "Reengineering a Surgical Service Line: Focusing on Core Process Improvement." *American Journal of Medical Quality* 12 (2): 120–29.

National Institute of Standards and Technology (NIST). 2006. "Baldrige National Quality Program Healthcare Criteria for Performance Excellence." [Online information; retrieved 1/2/06.] www. baldrige.gov/Criteria.htm.

Nelson, E. C., J. J. Mohr, P. B. Batalden, and S. K. Plume. 1996. "Improving Healthcare, Part 1: The Clinical Value Compass." *Joint Commission Journal on Quality Improvement* 22 (4): 243–58.

Wheeler, D. J. 2000. *Understanding Variation: The Key to Managing Chaos,*
    2nd edition. Knoxville, TN: SPC Press.
Zelman, W. N., D. Blazer, J. M. Glover, P. Bumgarner, and L. Cancilla. 1999.
    "Issues for Academic Health Centers to Consider Before Implementing a
    Balanced-Scorecard Effort." *Academic Medicine* 74 (12): 1269–77.

Exercise

Objective: To explore sources of comparative data.

Instructions

1. Go to the latest version of the "National Healthcare Quality Report":
    www.qualitytools.ahrq.gov/qualityreport/browse/browse.aspx.
2. For each of the four categories of measures (effectiveness, patient
    safety, timeliness, and patient centeredness), explore the links that
    explain the importance of the categories as well as the selected
    measures and/or the sources of the selected measures. List key
    points in the appropriate column on The National Healthcare
    Quality Report Worksheet below.
3. List those performance measures currently used in your own work set-
    ting that reflect your organization's performance in these categories.

The National Healthcare Quality Report Worksheet

	Key Points	**Specific Measures in my Work Setting**
Effectiveness (choose one condition)		
Patient Safety		
Timeliness		
Patient centeredness		

11

ORGANIZATIONAL TRACTION

Objectives

- To describe the elements of organizational traction
- To describe the importance of organizational traction in initiating and sustaining ongoing performance improvement
- To gain an appreciation for the need to define current reality

When an unexpected snow catches a warm-weather city by surprise, cars may be seen slipping and sliding on the roads. A bicyclist uses one type of bike for riding on the street and a different type for riding on mountain trails. A ski racer carefully chooses her wax to avoid being slowed down by the snow. A car hydroplanes on the highway during an intense rainstorm.

Each of these situations is influenced by traction. The ability to understand and manage traction is the difference between safely getting to work on time and sliding off the road, getting stuck in the mud and having a great ride, winning a ski race and losing it, and arriving safely at a destination and reeling out of control.

Traction is the force that allows something to stay connected to a surface. It may be intentionally increased to attach an object to the surface (e.g., with specially designed tires) or intentionally decreased to detach an object from the surface (e.g., with types of ski wax). The force of traction is also exerted when something is being drawn; pulleys, cranes, and winches enable a person to draw, lift, or move something that he would be unable to move otherwise. The same can be said of organizations. An understanding of organizational traction and organizational pulleys allows managers to initiate and sustain movement in quality, change, and performance improvement efforts and to stay the course toward the goal.

A common question that managers and students alike ask when discussing improvement efforts is, "How do you get people to change?" In his classic *Harvard Business Review* article, Frederick Herzberg (2003) introduces the phrase "KITA"—an acronym for "kick in the 'pants'." He offers KITA as one approach to motivating employees and job enrichment (i.e., designing meaningful work that employees desire to do) as another. To initiate or motivate organizational change, the manager may choose a push strategy, or the manager may choose strategies that manage traction in the work environment to draw employees along a path of change and improvement.

This chapter explores two types of organizational traction. The first type helps managers initiate change in much the same way traction is used to get a car going on a slippery surface rather than having it sit there spinning its wheels. The second type helps managers maintain an ongoing environment of quality and performance improvement—that is, once the car gets going, it has to be kept moving.

Initiating Change

The Animal Control Services team at a county health department recognized that the community had a huge problem. In the past several years, there had been an increase in county pet populations, stray animals, and animal bites. In addition, rabies had reemerged after the county had been rabies free for years. The team made some progress when it instituted a 100 percent sterilization requirement for adopted animals. Although the department offered pet sterilization to any animal currently being adopted, because the process was cumbersome, many owners did not follow up once they took their new pet home or decided against adopting altogether. The team had an idea to redesign the pet adoption process that would enable pets to be sterilized before they left the animal shelter rather than having the new owner assume the responsibility.

The challenge was that their new plan would require some allocation of funds from the county commissioners. The team realized the importance of this public health issue; however, they were faced with the problem of how to communicate their sense of urgency to an audience with little knowledge of the issue. Faced with only five minutes on the county commissioner's agenda, the team decided on the following approach: present the facts and share the vision of a successful program. The veterinarian director of the team started the presentation with the following:

> Start with one female dog.... [I]n the first year, she produces an average of eight puppies, four of them females...in the second year, production of first and second generation females is 40 pups, 20 of them females...in the third year, production from three generations of females is 200 pups...in the fourth year, production from four generations is 1,000...and so on.... [B]y the eighth generation, this one female pup has resulted in the production of 625,000 puppies!!! (McNeil et al. 2002).

After the veterinarian gave a few statistics on animal bites and rabies and a brief overview of the plan for the new pet adoption process, the county commissioners were sold. A local reporter concluded a column describing the Animal Control Services's proposal with this comment: "The only question at this point would seem to be, is it possible to move faster?" (*Wilmington Morning Star* 2002).

Animal Control Services understood how to use traction to engage stakeholders, gain support for its vision, and jump-start its improvement effort. First, it stated the facts, which in this case were the reproductive capacity of one female puppy and the health consequences of pet over-population. Next, it offered its vision of a process. Finally, by clearly revealing the performance gap between what currently existed and what was possible, the team used the concept of creative tension to establish the traction needed to get its effort moving forward (McNeil et al. 2002).

Creative Tension

Just as the medical specialty of surgery consists of such subspecialties as neurosurgery, orthopedic surgery, and plastic surgery, the field of systems thinking also consists of subfields. One of these subfields is called "structural dynamics." Tension resolution is the fundamental building block in structural dynamics (Fritz 1996). When a difference exists between one thing and another, the resulting discrepancy creates the tendency toward movement. One type of tension found in organizations is called "creative tension," which is formed by the discrepancy between an organization's current level of performance and its desired level and vision for the future.

The rubber-band metaphor has been used to illustrate the concept of creative tension (Senge 1990). Think of holding a rubber band, with one end in each hand and one hand above the other. Stretch the rubber band, and feel the tension of the pull. Think of the higher hand as vision—that is, the desired future state of the organization. Think of the lower hand as current reality—that is, the current level of the organization's performance. The tension may be released from the rubber band by only three ways.

The first way to relieve tension is to let go of the end clasped by the lower hand. As the tension is released, the rubber band is drawn to the top hand. The greater the tension, the faster and more strongly the rubber band will return to the top hand. In organizations, this tension resolution may be seen as drawing the organization toward a vision. The second way to relieve tension is to let go of the end clasped by the higher hand. As the tension is released, the rubber band is drawn to the bottom hand. In organizations, this tension resolution may be seen as simply maintaining the status quo or stagnating performance, despite well-intentioned efforts to improve. The third way to relieve tension is by stretching the rubber band beyond its natural limit and breaking it. In organizations, this type of tension resolution may be seen in situations where too much is expected, too fast, and without adequate resources; as a result, people and processes "break." Symptoms of this last type of tension resolution include employee turnover, morale problems, poor performance, and medical errors.

When organizational change and performance are viewed through a systems perspective, tension resolution is the key traction tool for changing behavior. The essential elements for creative tension to be present in an organization are current reality, vision, and an actual or perceived gap between the two. The manager's role is to consciously generate, make visible, and regulate creative tension in the organization to leverage the resulting tendency toward movement (Senge 1990; Heifetz and Laurie 2001).

Current Reality

Establishing creative tension requires some sort of common, objective description of current reality. The description may range from a very simple evaluation to an in-depth organizational assessment. Without some objective depiction of the current situation of the organization, individuals may be left to create their own pictures of current reality based on their own limited information sets. Without a shared understanding of current reality, the manager's ability to take advantage of creative tension is limited.

Organizational assessment and diagnosis may be more familiar to strategic planners who have used SWOT (strengths, weaknesses, opportunities, threats) or PEST (political, economic, social, technological) analyses or to organizational development professionals than to managers. However, the concept and practice of assessment offer a valuable way for managers to document, communicate, and promote a shared understanding of current reality. An organizational assessment or self-assessment simply refers to a systematic or repeatable method of examining the organization for its strengths and performance gaps. An organizational self-assessment conducted at regular intervals (e.g., annually, biannually) provides managers with the opportunity and impetus to systematically reexamine, document, and communicate current reality relative to desired organizational activities, strategies, and performance results. In Chapter 5, several systems models are introduced, including the BNQP Healthcare Criteria for Performance Excellence. The Baldrige model may be best known for its national award, but it is also an important guide for organizational self-assessment.

As managers begin to understand creative tension, they will also begin to see that a performance measurement system is a vital management tool to describe, monitor, and communicate current reality. In the absence of performance measures, those within the organization will define current reality on the basis of their own mental models, knowledge, and previous experiences. As a result, some may hold an overly positive view of the organization's current reality, and others may hold a disproportionately negative view. The net effect is the absence of a shared understanding of current reality and no shared understanding of the performance gap, which is necessary for creative tension. Without creative tension, there is no need for tension resolution and, in turn, no traction for change.

Vision

Vision plays a role in leadership (Kotter 2001; Kouzes and Posner 2002; Tichey 1997), personal effectiveness (Covey 1990), organizational effectiveness (Senge 1990), art (Fritz 1989), and even survival (Frankl 1962). Vision is also an essential element in creative tension and, thus, in creating traction for change.

Visions may be found at a variety of levels within healthcare. The Office of Disease Prevention and Health Promotion, through the U.S. Department of Health and Human Services's Healthy People Initiatives, offers an overall vision for the nation's health: "[R]egardless of age, gender, race or ethnicity, income, education, geographic location, disability, and sexual orientation—every person in every community across the Nation deserves equal access to comprehensive, culturally competent, community-based healthcare systems that are committed to serving the needs of the individual and promoting community health" (Healthy People 2010 2005a).

This vision provides a common direction for diverse groups that share the interest of improving health and healthcare within the United States. The vision is further described by defining specific areas of focus, such as access, environmental health, public health infrastructure, and infectious diseases, and by defining ideal performance in a variety of health indicators. The ten health indicators—physical activity, overweight and obesity, tobacco use, substance abuse, responsible sexual behavior, mental health, injury and violence, environmental quality, immunization, and access to healthcare—provide direction for groups to individualize their own community visions within the larger national context (Healthy People 2010 2005b).

Organizations often have an overall vision for the future. Managers may also use the concept of vision in a variety of ways and at various levels within the organization. Managers may have visions for their careers, for their own professional contribution to quality healthcare, or for their ideal departments or service areas. Managers may ask a team to describe its ideal vision for a particular work process or process of care. When managers understand that vision is an essential element of creative tension, they will also realize that vision is essential to quality management and organizational effectiveness.

In creating a vision, it is helpful to describe characteristics of the ideal future state. Questions that physicians may pose when creating a vision for their own office practice may include the following:

If my practice were recognized as one of the best in the country,

- What would patients and families say about the care they received?
- What would patients and families say about their interactions with me? With my office staff?
- What would my colleagues around the country say about my practice?
- What processes in my office would colleagues most want to emulate?

In addition, physicians may want to consider these questions:

- How do I and my office staff feel after a day's work?

- If a prominent journal or newspaper were writing about my office practice, what would the article say?

When creating a vision, one should not be limited by what is possible or what is not possible. By defining characteristics of the ideal future rather than ideal interventions, a manager may balance describing an ideal future with present constraints. Healthcare workers often respond with "We would have that new computer system" or "We would totally remodel the office" when asked about their ideal unit or office. However, financial constraints may not allow for these expenditures at the time, which makes constructing the vision an exercise in futility rather than a chance to describe a future ideal state. Rather than "We would have that new computer system," the ideal answer might be, "We have streamlined, user-friendly documentation and communication mechanisms in place to provide needed information for safe care, efficient internal office operations, and patient education." Rather than "We would totally remodel the office," the ideal answer might be, "Patients will find a clean, accessible, comfortable, and relaxing office environment that respects their privacy and confidentiality."

By defining characteristics of the ideal future rather than ideal interventions that are more specific to the way things are now, opportunities for finding creative and flexible ways of achieving the vision while working within the constraints of the situation may be enhanced.

Maintaining an Ongoing Environment of Quality and Performance Improvement

In Chapter 7, the concept of mental models is introduced as a deeply ingrained way of thinking that influences how a person sees and understands the world and how a person acts. Context is a concept closely related to mental models and is defined as "the unquestioning assumptions through which all experience is filtered" (Davis 1982, 26). In this book, the term "mental models" refer to an individual's assumptions, and the term "context" refers to organizational assumptions that guide how the organization defines itself and how it operates.

Context

Two illustrations of context may be explored to better understand the subtle difference between mental models and context. Here is the first illustration.

> Consider this analogy. You inherit your grandmother's house. Unknown to you is one peculiarity: all the light fixtures have bulbs that give off a blue rather than yellow light. You find that you don't like the feel of the rooms and spend a lot of time and money repainting walls, reupholstering furniture, and replacing carpets. You never seem to get it quite right, but nonetheless, you

rationalize that at least it is improving with each thing you do. Then one day you notice the blue light bulbs and change them. Suddenly, all that you fixed is broken.

Context is like the color of the light, not the objects in the room. Context colors everything in the corporation. More accurately, the context alters what we see, usually without our being aware of it (Goss, Pascale, and Athos 1993, 99–100).

An external community focus may represent one operating context for a healthcare organization, while an internal organizational focus may represent a different operating context. A focus on improving the quality of health services delivered may represent one operating context, while a focus on improving health of the community is another. Management decisions about resource allocation, prevention, or continuum-of-care issues will differ depending on the context or assumptions about the organization's focus or role in the community.

Consider this second illustration of context, which suggests a corollary to the concept: content.

Most parents have dreams for their children. Some want their children to be doctors, some musicians, and all want them to be healthy, wealthy, and wise. These are parents raising their children by focusing on content. Following in a father's footsteps, or in the footsteps father never had and therefore wants for his son, [is a] well-known example of this approach. Other parents, however, raise their children by focusing on context. In Helen Keller's famous phrase, their dream is, "be all you can be." The orientation here is to "parent" the context and let the child discover the content (Davis 1982, 28).

As stated in the illustration, managers may also find themselves facing the dichotomy of which—context or content—to manage. One may think of the distinctions between context and content as they are demonstrated in Figure 10.3. The boundary of the circle is the context; the inside of the circle is the content (Davis 1982).

Historically, healthcare managers have been promoted on the basis of their content expertise: an excellent pharmacist becomes the manager of the entire pharmacy department; an excellent engineer becomes the manager of the facilities maintenance department; or an excellent clinician becomes a department, division, or unit manager. These managerial roles generally include direct supervision of both the people and the work.

Today, the organizations, environments, processes, and technologies in healthcare are so complex that managers cannot be experts on managing and on the content of the work that needs to be managed. Managers' roles will increasingly move away from managing content to managing context. This means employees with fundamental knowledge of the work itself will carry out and improve their work processes, while managers will ensure that employees have the appropriate tools, information, knowledge, and competency to effectively do their jobs and deliver quality services and products.

Managing context also suggests managing the boundaries of the system, which may be a unit, a department, an office practice, a service line, or an entire organization. Boundaries may be defined in terms of scope of work, decision-making authority, or accountability. The manager may set or reset the boundaries on the basis of environmental conditions and other organizational considerations. In a department with a high ratio of experienced employees, the manager may expand the boundary so that staff are more autonomous in their decision making. However, in a department composed of a young or inexperienced staff, the manager may tighten the boundaries of decision making until staff gains knowledge, ability, and confidence in their own decision-making skills.

Managing the boundaries of the system also suggests that the managers not only define their own areas of responsibility but also the interfaces that occur at the boundaries. As healthcare organizations become more complex and teams are increasingly used to accomplish the organization's work, the supervisory role also shifts to one of "boundary manager" (Orsburn et al. 1990). This means that, rather than supervising individuals, the supervisor helps teams interact with each other as needed to coordinate work, communicate information, or resolve problems. Likewise, effectively managing context requires an awareness and understanding of the interfaces with other systems both within and outside of the organization. In the trade-offs example described in Chapter 4, the manager who anticipated unintended consequences of reducing hospital length of stay and proactively worked with the nursing homes demonstrated an awareness and understanding of the interface between acute care and nursing home care.

The best way to become aware of context and then draw the appropriate boundary for the system is by asking the right questions (Davis 1982). For managers, the key to asking the right questions is not to be afraid to challenge current assumptions; otherwise, the answers to the questions will simply be a restatement of what is already known rather than a way to truly seek to understand and explore what is beyond the current boundary of knowledge or awareness. The importance of challenging assumptions may be seen in the ambulatory surgery improvement example referred to in chapters 5 and 9. The prevailing assumption at the time was to use restructuring to reduce costs; specifically, the organization reduces the number of registered nurse (RN) positions by eliminating RNs or replacing them with unlicensed personnel (Gordon 2005). In the ambulatory surgery example, "because the outcome of cost savings and value had been defined at the onset of the project in terms of length of stay and total consumption of resources, not just in terms of staffing mix, cost savings [were] realized despite a predominantly RN staff" (Kelly et al. 1997, 126). By replacing the assumption that restructuring was the only solution with a principles-driven change process, this team was able to improve throughput, reduce costs, maintain clinical outcomes, and improve patient satisfaction while retaining RNs in their care-delivery model, an approach "quite different from the trend of decreasing professional staff and increasing mix of unlicensed support personnel" (Kelly et al. 1997, 128).

Without skills in challenging and managing context, the ability of managers and other healthcare professionals to create and implement innovative improvements and attain excellent performance in healthcare systems will be limited. For this reason, the common theme of Section III in this book is to offer managers structured ways to test underlying assumptions and ask new questions about goals, purpose, measurement, implementation, and teams.

Context and Vision

A common cliché in healthcare is "change is a given," and the same can be said of ambiguity. Ambiguity and uncertainty will continue to increase as inherent characteristics of the environments in which healthcare organizations operate. Understanding the roles of vision and context can help managers create supportive work environments in the presence of ambiguity and uncertainty rather than chaotic and unstable environments.

A young child putting together a puzzle illustrates how vision and context are related. The child empties the puzzle pieces from the box and then props up the box to see a picture of what the puzzle is supposed to look like when it is completed. He then sorts the pieces: one group contains pieces with a straight edge or a corner shape, and one group contains the odd shapes. When asked why, the child replies, "To make the outside first." Once the outer edge of the puzzle is assembled, he goes about fitting in the rest of the pieces, knowing that each piece will eventually have its own place in the picture.

The manager's role in establishing vision may be thought of as making sure everyone in the organization has the ability to see the entire picture—that is, what the puzzle will look like when it is completed. The manager's role in setting the boundaries or context of the system may be thought of as putting together the outer edge of the puzzle. The images or shapes of the individual pieces may be thought of as the content, which is what goes on or what is done within the organization. Although there is much ambiguity at first about where the individual pieces should go, enough information is available to continue the task of building the puzzle or, in the manager's case, moving toward the vision of the future.

Conclusion

The key to sustainable change in organizations is to identify and address underlying structures, as described in Chapter 7. The key to initiating movement toward improvement is to address tension resolution. The key to maintaining an environment of ongoing performance improvement is to address context. These three activities fall within the manager's domain of responsibility; addressing the content—the actual care, work, and technical process—falls within the domain of responsibility of the frontline workers and care providers.

In clinical services, a physical examination or annual checkup is a commonplace activity. The exercise at the end of this chapter continues to explore the value of an organizational assessment in defining current reality by comparing it to a physical examination. Once the concept of traction is understood, the focus of implementing changes and improvements shifts from overcoming staff resistance to supporting staff success. Chapter 12 describes several implementation lessons that may enhance a manager's ability to support staff and, in turn, successfully integrate improvements into operations of the organization.

Companion Readings

Davis, S. M. 1982. "Transforming Organizations: The Key to Strategy Is Context." *Organizational Dynamics* 10 (3): 64–80.

Heifetz, R. A., and D. L. Laurie. 2001. "The Work of Leadership." *Harvard Business Review* 79 (11): 131–40.

References

Covey, S. R. 1990. *The Seven Habits of Highly Effective People*. New York: Simon and Schuster.

Davis, S. M. 1982. "Transforming Organizations: The Key to Strategy Is Context." *Organizational Dynamics* 10 (3): 64–80.

Frankl, V. E. 1962. *Man's Search for Meaning: An Introduction to Logotherapy*. Boston: Beacon Press.

Fritz, R. 1989. *The Path of Least Resistance: Learning to Become the Creative Force in Your Own Life*. New York: Ballantine.

———. 1996. *Corporate Tides: The Inescapable Laws of Organizational Structure*. San Francisco: Berrett-Koehler Publishers.

Gordon, S. 2005. *Nursing Against the Odds: How Health Care Cost Cutting, Media Stereotypes, and Medical Hubris Undermine Nurses and Patient Care*. Ithaca, NY: Cornell University Press.

Goss, T., R. Pascale, and A. Athos. 1993. "The Reinvention Roller Coaster: Risking the Present for a Powerful Future." *Harvard Business Review* 71 (6): 97–108.

Healthy People 2010. 2005a. "A Systematic Approach to Health Improvement: Objectives." [Online information; retrieved 12/05/05.] www.health.gov/healthypeople/Document/html/uih/uih_2.htm#obj.

———. 2005b. "What Are the Leading Indicators?" [Online information; retrieved 12/05/05.] www.healthypeople.gov/LHI/lhiwhat.htm.

Heifetz, R. A., and D. L. Laurie. 2001. "The Work of Leadership." *Harvard Business Review* 79 (11): 131–40.

Herzberg, F. 2003. "One More Time: How Do You Motivate Employees?" *Harvard Business Review* 81 (1): 87–96.

Kelly, D. L., S. L. Pestotnik, M. C. Coons, and J. W. Lelis. 1997. "Reengineering a Surgical Service Line: Focusing on Core Process Improvement." *American Journal of Medical Quality* 12 (2): 120–29.

Kotter, J. P. 2001. "What Leaders Really Do." *Harvard Business Review* 79 (11): 85–90.

Kouzes, J. M., and B. Z. Posner. 2002. *The Leadership Challenge, 3rd edition.* San Francisco: Jossey-Bass.

McNeil, J. P., D. Brown, D. Howard, B. McClure, and G. R. Weedon. 2002. "Sterilization Protects Animals and You." Presentation to the University of North Carolina at Chapel Hill Management Academy for Public Health, April 25.

Orsburn, J. D., L. Moran, E. Musselwhite, and J. H. Zenger. 1990. *Self-Directed Work Teams: The New American Challenge.* Homewood, IL: Business One Irwin.

Senge, P. M. 1990. *The Fifth Discipline: The Art and Practice of the Learning Organization.* New York: Doubleday Currency.

Tichey, N. M. 1997. *The Leadership Engine: How Winning Companies Build Leaders at Every Level.* New York: Harper Collins Publishers.

Wilmington Morning Star. 2002. "Saving Pets and Taxpayers." (January 7): 6A.

Exercise

Objective: To gain an appreciation for a regular assessment of current reality in an organization.

Instructions

1. An integral activity in any healthcare provider–patient encounter involves the physical examination, checkup, or assessment. This exercise will examine what may be learned about the organizational examination, checkup, or assessment from this routine clinical practice.

   For questions 1a through 1e, you may choose to record your responses on the Assessment Worksheet below or one similar to it.

   a. Describe the purpose of an annual physical examination. You may answer from a provider or patient point of view. You may discuss a physical examination, a well-child checkup, or even a dental appointment.

b. Describe the general sequence of events that occur during this examination.

c. How do you (if you answered as a provider) or the provider (if you answered as a patient) know what to do to complete the examination?

d. Describe why the examination is done in this particular way.

e. Answer the same questions for an organization, and fill in the "Organizational Checkup" column in the worksheet below.

f. On the basis of your responses to the above questions, describe why managers should or should not perform organizational checkups on a routine basis.

Assessment Worksheet

	Physical Checkup	Organizational Checkup
Purpose		
Sequence of events		
How do you know what to do?		
Why is it done this way?		

IMPLEMENTATION LESSONS

Objective

- To address operational considerations related to implementing improvements
- To introduce an implementation framework for managers
- To gain an appreciation for the influence of mental models on implementation

Consider two approaches to purchasing a new home. Every day for a week, Person A searches the real-estate advertisements in the newspapers. Her diligent search yields some properties that she is interested in, so she calls a realtor for a tour of each. After seeing a certain property, she immediately knows this is her perfect house. The realtor refers her to a mortgage company to work out the financing. Person A is confident that no problem will arise because, based on her own calculations, her salary will cover the monthly payments. But then she receives the bad news: she does not qualify for the financing. Payments on a new car bought six months earlier, outstanding credit card bills from a recent vacation, and a small savings account all work against her. Person A only qualifies for a loan that is much smaller than she had anticipated and needs for her dream home.

Person A's coworker, Person B, has a hobby of scanning the real-estate news. For years, Person B has been watching trends, and so she has identified a particular area of the city in which she would like to purchase a house. Based on the average housing prices in that area, Person B calculates what she will need for a down payment as well as for monthly mortgage payments. She systematically accumulates the funds for the down payment, makes sure she pays her credit card balances down to zero every month, and prequalifies with a mortgage company. Although most of her friends and coworkers drive new cars, her car is five years old but completely paid for. When Person B's "perfect house" comes on the market, she is the first to see it and is able to complete the purchase without a problem. When Person A overhears Person B talking about her new address, Person A cannot believe it; she wonders, "How could she possibly afford that place when she makes the same salary as I do?"

The answer to Person A's question is that these coworkers used two entirely different approaches to planning and implementing their processes for house buying. Person A used an approach called "forward planning," which involves taking one step at a time and not knowing the next step until after the previous step is completed. Person B used an approach called "reverse planning" (Dorner 1996), which involves defining the desired end result—in this case, her ideal house—and then working backward to determine a practical or logical starting point to the step-by-step process of getting to the end result. In reverse planning, each step is a necessary precondition to the next step. By planning in this manner, Person B could make purposeful choices (e.g., not buying a new car, reducing her credit card debt) that would help her toward, rather than become barriers to, the end goal of purchasing her ideal house.

Similar approaches have been described in the literature. Habit number two in *The Seven Habits of Highly Effective People* by Stephen Covey (1990) advises to "begin with the end in mind." The "solution after next principle," from *Breakthrough Thinking: The Seven Principles of Creative Problem Solving,* indicates that more effective solutions may be generated "by working backward from an ideal target solution for the future" (Nadler and Hibino 1994).

This chapter introduces an implementation framework derived from the common themes of these three approaches. First, however, operational considerations for implementing improvement efforts are described and the manager's role in supporting team success as well as the relationship between mental models and successful implementation are explored.

Operational Considerations

In addition to the particulars of the intended intervention, managers should take into account the measurement system, unintended consequences, and staff issues when planning for the implementation of an improvement or change effort.

Measurement System

"How will you know if the change is an improvement?" (Langley et al. 1996) is a fundamental question managers should ask about any improvement effort. Chapter 8 illustrates an example of how a surgical services manager first set general goals to be able to establish overall direction and specific goals. The manager's first goal was to design and implement the performance measurement system. This goal took a while to achieve because data had to be collected from a variety of sources and from different electronic databases, but it taught the manager the importance of having a measurement system in place as the foundation for understanding the impact of future interventions, whether for a specific process improvement (e.g., preoperative laboratory tests) or for an intervention affecting the entire department (e.g., redesigned governance structure) (Kelly et al. 1997).

Managers must be able to distinguish between measuring the impact of a single intervention and measuring the overall performance of the system (e.g., department, service, organization) over which the manager is responsible. Unlike a clinical trial, where the researchers are closely manipulating the variables to be tested, the numerous interrelated variables at work in complex healthcare organizations make it difficult for managers to determine the precise impact of a single intervention. The characteristics of dynamic complexity (see Chapter 4) and the subsequent need to use multiple goals when operating in complex systems (see Chapter 8) suggest that measures of a single change are only one component of an overall performance measurement system.

A performance measurement system should be the very first step of implementation, not only because of its role in describing, monitoring, and communicating current reality and progress toward the vision (see Chapter 11) but also because it provides feedback about the influence of improvement interventions on the behavior of the overall system. If a measurement system is already in place, then the manager/team/organization may continue with implementing operational and other improvements. Although not typically thought of as an implementation intervention, managers may view implementing or improving the current performance measurement system as a quality intervention within the management domain.

If the manager does not already have an effective performance measurement system in place, planning other improvements may continue; however, implementation should be delayed until the measurement system is designed and put into place. If customer and stakeholder requirements are drivers of improvement, the general direction of performance requirements should be known, and general rather than specific performance goals may be set initially. In other words, the manager desires some area of performance to improve, and the improvement may be measured by an indicator going down (e.g., costs or cycle times) or going up (e.g., patient satisfaction). Once a means to measure the impact of the intervention is in place, managers or teams may implement the intervention and monitor the direction of performance in relation to the goal. As ongoing data are collected and thus provide specific feedback about performance, more specific goals may be set.

This approach to measurement may sound counterintuitive to those accustomed to measurement within the context of clinical research or other approaches that require accumulating baseline data trends over time. Derived from a management and performance improvement mental model on measurement, the performance measurement approach described in the preceding paragraph takes into account the nature of healthcare organizations as complex systems and offers managers a way to reduce the improvement-process cycle time, which is the time from when the improvement is initiated to the time when results are seen. Note that management data must demonstrate reliability and validity; however, because the intended use is to gather feedback about the system's behavior and monitor and improve performance, other data characteristics (e.g., sample size, bias definition, data-collection methods, the relationship of the data to the hypothesis) may differ from data used for other purposes (James 2001).

Unintended Consequences

In a large tertiary care hospital, one improvement effort was aimed at decreasing the amount of time patients spent on a ventilator after coronary bypass surgery. A patient's progress toward recovery could be greatly enhanced if less time was spent connected to a ventilator. The improvement team thoughtfully took into account the upstream influences on the patient recovery process by inviting operating room staff and an anesthesiologist to be members of the improvement team.

After bypass surgery, when a patient met the required clinical criteria, she was transferred from the ICU to the acute care patient-care unit. After the new ICU protocol was put into place, patients who had coronary bypass surgery began arriving in the acute care unit a day earlier and were sicker than before. Although these patients were not on ventilators anymore, the extra day of recovery made a difference in other aspects of their care. The acute care unit was finding itself short staffed on numerous occasions. Although the same number of nurses was being scheduled, the higher patient acuity, requiring more intense nursing care, led to the unit's understaffing.

After several weeks, the nurses in the acute care unit realized that a change had been made in the ICU's postoperative process. It took the nurse manager several months to hire the required staff to meet the new acuity demands, during which time the existing nurses remained short staffed and overworked.

Chapter 10 introduces the concept of unintended consequences, which are important considerations for managers and teams when implementing improvement efforts within their own work areas, departments, and organizations. Anticipating, identifying, measuring, and proactively managing unintended consequences should be considered in any implementation plan. Figure 12.1 illustrates how this ICU improvement team might have identified unintended consequences by asking not only "Who affects our process" but also "Who is affected by our process?"

Managers' Role in Team Success

Successful implementation actually begins when an improvement effort is initiated. While the team is responsible for designing and implementing improvements, the manager is responsible for creating the conditions that will enable the team to succeed. The conditions may be thought of in terms of the phases of the team's activities: beginning the process, designing the actual improvement, and putting the improvements into place.

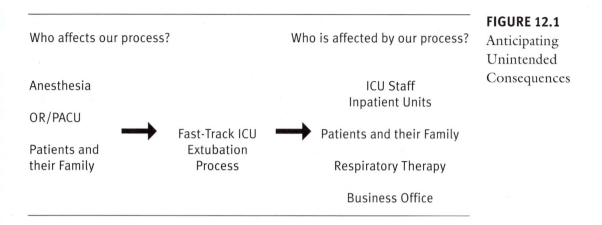

FIGURE 12.1
Anticipating
Unintended
Consequences

Who affects our process?   Who is affected by our process?

Anesthesia   ICU Staff
                                                         Inpatient Units
OR/PACU
                          Fast-Track ICU   Patients and their Family
Patients and   Extubation
their Family   Process   Respiratory Therapy

                                                        Business Office

Beginning the Process

To enhance team success, the manager must provide the team with a clear understanding of what it has been organized to do (purpose) and a clear direction (goals). The managers should attend to four additional tasks at the beginning of an improvement effort: define participant accountabilities, establish boundaries, communicate managerial expectations, and promote buy-in.

First, the accountabilities of all participants should be clearly defined. Accountabilities may include how decisions will be made or what type of participation is expected from members of the team (e.g., attendance). Defining accountabilities does not necessarily mean that the manager makes all the rules; rather, he or she ensures that the rules are clearly defined. For example, when one administrator asked surgeons how they would like to be involved in an upcoming improvement effort to address patient flow in the preoperative area, the surgeons indicated that they would prefer to have a proposed plan presented at their monthly medical staff meetings. They would then provide feedback and recommendations through their already established governance structure. They did not have the time or desire to be involved in the day-to-day details of designing the improvements, but they definitely wanted to be part of the process of evaluating and refining proposed solutions.

Second, managers should clearly define the boundaries of what can and cannot be changed—that is, what aspects of the problem, solution, or process are negotiable and not negotiable. For example, the improvement team of an emergency department was told to think "outside the box." However, when the team presented its outside-the-box and very expensive idea to hospital administration, the team was told that the idea was impossible to implement because of the associated expense. The lack of boundaries, rather than spurring creativity, ended up demoralizing the team members and discouraging them from continuing to participate in this or future improvement efforts. The morale and engagement of the team members could have been preserved had the manager defined the boundaries for the team, by indicating, for example, the maximum dollars available for remodeling or new equipment, very early in the improvement effort.

Third, if an improvement team needs to deliver specific results or follow specific constraints, these expectations should be clearly defined and communicated at the onset of any change or improvement effort. Expectations may include timelines (e.g., within a certain operating budget cycle), results (e.g., improve cycle times by 5 percent), or budgets (e.g., dollars or time allotted for project team meetings).

Finally, to promote staff buy-in, the manager should "sell the problem, not the solution" (Bridges 1991). When employees are informed about the nature and consequences of the problem, they are much more likely to be open to various solutions designed to improve it.

Managers should also be careful to build on the current strengths and accomplishments of their staff. If not introduced tactfully, an improvement effort may send the unintended message that employees are not doing a good job. For example, a manager began a new position at a state health department after working for many years in a hospital that had been recognized for its quality-improvement efforts. This manager had been recruited to help the health department improve its work processes to become more efficient. As the manager became acquainted with the department, she realized that the focus on efficiency was a response to major budget cuts in the recent legislative session. As she introduced her goals of improved efficiency to employees in the department, she first acknowledged the successful programs that the department had designed and implemented. She then educated the employees about specific changes in the environment and stakeholder requirements. To respond to these changing external factors, the department needed to evaluate and adapt its internal operations. Next, she explained that to preserve funds for the department programs, the department needed to become more efficient and productive in how they administered these programs.

Designing the Improvement

Throughout the course of an improvement effort, the manager should provide an opportunity for team members to interact with each other and with others in the organization. When thinking about the composition of a project team, participants from outside the manager's own scope of responsibility should be considered if they have fundamental knowledge of the process targeted for improvement. For example, a team organized to improve discharge planning in an inpatient surgical unit in a large hospital included not only nurses from this unit but also nurses from "upstream care" (e.g., operating room and intensive care unit) and non-nursing providers (e.g., dietitian, social worker, and respiratory therapist). In this way the team integrated all of the aspects and sources of care the patients received during their hospital stay into the discharge planning process.

The manager is instrumental in ensuring access to the information the team needs to effectively study and improve the problem. Information may come in many forms, including management reports, clinical data, and regulatory requirements. Managers may also assist teams by providing access to information that the team may not know is available. For example, one manager helped a team organize a discussion with several internal customers so that they could better understand their customers' perspective. Another manager helped link a team with the organization's corporate marketing department, which in turn invited the team members to observe a patient focus group. This manager also helped the team to schedule the hospital administrator to come to one of their meetings to answer questions and address concerns.

Putting the Improvements in Place

The manager's responsibility is to ensure that the appropriate organizational conditions are in place to enhance successful implementation. Managers may do this by asking themselves the question, "What needs to happen to ensure success?" The following considerations serve as starting points.

First, depending on the scope of the improvement effort, the manager may need to provide a staffing "cushion," which means that he or she has to overstaff initially. Adapting to something new and learning new processes or roles takes time and planning ahead; the manager must not only acknowledge but also actively support the staff's learning curves. Second, the manager may need to negotiate for the necessary short-term budget or productivity variances required for the transition period; however, the long-term benefits to productivity should compensate for the short-term variance. Third, managers must also ask, "Do staff members have the knowledge and skills required to succeed?" The manager, again, is responsible for ensuring that all staff have the necessary information, training, and tools to enable them to successfully implement improvements. No matter how elegant the solution, inadequately prepared staff can undermine the success of implementation.

Relationship Between Mental Models and Implementation

Although a cliché, the phrase "actions speak louder than words" represents an important consideration when implementing improvement efforts. The idea is also captured in the phrase, "Process and content are inseparable" (Kofman and Senge 1993, 19). This concept means that how a manager goes about improving is equally as important as what the manager chooses to improve.

The term "content" refers to an actual intervention, technique, or process improvement. The term "process" refers to all of the steps involved in

- identifying, studying, and evaluating a problem;
- initiating, organizing, selecting, and facilitating the solution-generating process;
- communicating and preparing staff to implement the intervention; and
- measuring, evaluating, refining, and sustaining performance.

Setting effective goals and clarifying purpose guide managers and teams in content decisions to improve performance results. An awareness of the influence of mental models guides managers in process decisions to improve implementation results.

As described in Chapter 7, mental models shape an individual's actions, and likewise, an individual's actions provide clues to the underlying mental models. For example, a manager who talks about empowerment but holds tightly to decisions and information sends the message through his actions that he does not promote empowerment. Management interventions and change processes may also be considered activities that provide clues to underlying mental models and that, in turn, send messages to staff. An improvement team may be told to "share opinions openly" or that "all opinions are welcome." However, if team members are rebuked each time a contrasting idea is offered, the team quickly realizes that the process is operating from a mental model that in fact does not welcome all opinions.

The exercise at the end of the chapter provides readers with the opportunity to explore the relationship between mental models and implementation in more depth.

Framework for Implementation

Figure 12.2 illustrates a conceptual framework for implementation, referred to in this book as breakthrough vision, incremental implementation (Kelly et al. 1997).

Similar diagrams resembling a flight of stairs have been used to illustrate the incremental nature of continuous improvement of existing technology compared with breakthrough technologies. Figure 12.3 shows an example of how the writing process has improved over time, beginning with paper-and-pen approaches on the left, followed by incremental improvements to paper-and-pen methods. The first large step represents the invention of the typewriter (A), which is then followed by additional improvements to the typewriter (B). The second large step represents the breakthrough technology of computerized word processing (C).

A challenge for healthcare managers is that breakthrough technologies are most often associated with clinical breakthroughs in diagnosis (e.g., magnetic resonance imaging), intervention (e.g., minimally invasive surgery techniques), treatment (e.g., new drugs), or prevention (e.g., polio vaccination). Although specific technology breakthroughs are available that may enhance performance in the management domain (e.g., electronic

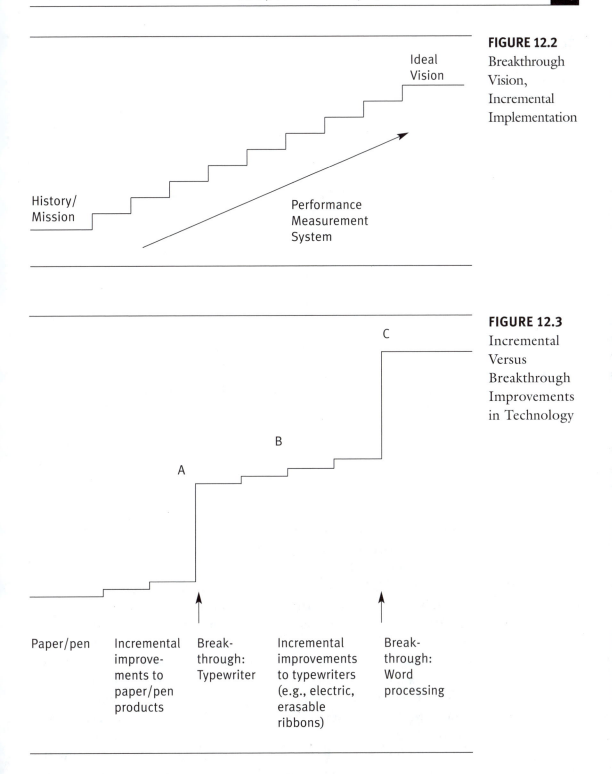

FIGURE 12.2
Breakthrough
Vision,
Incremental
Implementation

FIGURE 12.3
Incremental
Versus
Breakthrough
Improvements
in Technology

information systems), management breakthroughs that influence organizational performance are most often associated with the environment in which the clinical technologies may be used. Management breakthroughs may be seen in (1) areas such as philosophies, approaches, and tools that

FIGURE 12.4
Refining
Vision/
Context as
Management
Breakthroughs

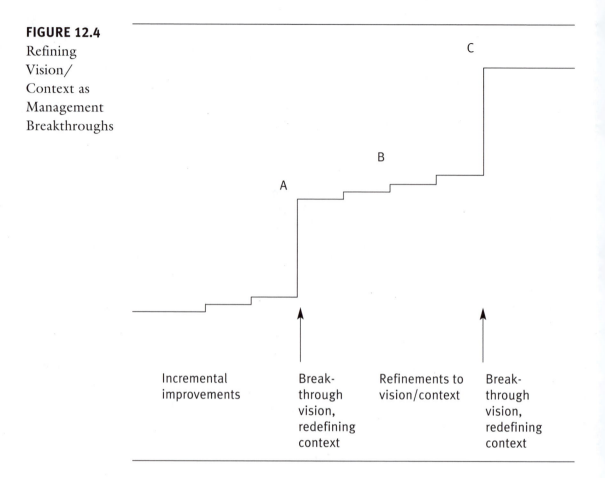

FIGURE 12.4
Refining
Vision/
Context as
Management
Breakthroughs

enable managers to promote innovations in the operating environment and (2) work processes that enable patients to fully realize the benefit of advancements in clinical technology.

Figure 12.4 illustrates the assumptions on which the breakthrough vision, incremental implementation framework is based. Rather than the breakthrough resulting from a technical invention, the breakthrough is defined through the vision and/or context of the department, service, or organization (A). Refinements or adjustments may be made according to changes in the environment or customer/stakeholder expectations (B). The vision and/or context may require fundamental redefinition periodically to stay current with changes in the larger operating environment (C).

The top stair in Figure 12.2 (upper right corner) represents the breakthrough vision and is labeled as the "ideal vision" of overall performance. The ideal vision may stretch as far as needed to illuminate the performance gap and thus establish creative tension (see Chapter 11). The bottom stair (lower left corner) is labeled "history/mission." Understanding the history of the organization, department, service, or technology helps

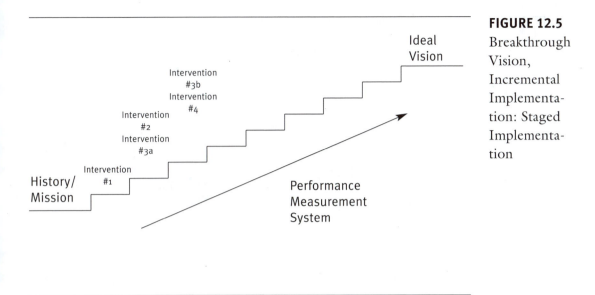

FIGURE 12.5

Breakthrough Vision, Incremental Implementation: Staged Implementation

managers identify and uncover issues, attitudes, or past events that may undermine implementation. An understanding of the past also promotes buy-in to change by grounding the change efforts through establishing continuity with past events (see Chapter 7). A clear statement of mission describes the purpose and justifies the existence of an organization, department, service, or process (see Chapter 9).

Connecting the bottom stair (history/mission) with the top stair (ideal vision) are numerous steps that represent specific interventions or improvements that are designed to move performance closer to the ideal. The steps taken toward achieving the vision must not be so great that they distract the care providers' focus and attention and place patient safety and outcomes at risk (Reason 1990). However, the steps taken in implementation must be large enough so that slipping back to the previous way of doing things is not possible. A step may have only one intervention, or several concurrent interventions may exist at a step. Some interventions may be completed quickly, and others may be broken down and achieved in several sequential steps, as shown in Figure 12.5. The diagonal line beneath the steps and pointing toward the ideal vision is labeled "Performance Measurement System," indicating that progress toward the vision is continually evaluated.

Figure 12.6 illustrates how the surgical services manager described in Chapter 8 implemented the unit's multiple goals in staged fashion according to this framework. The bottom step represents the mission of the service line. The top step on the right of the diagram represents the overall vision and the general goals. The performance measurement system is shown beneath the stairs and was the first intervention implemented. The first four

FIGURE 12.6
Breakthrough
Vision,
Incremental
Implementa-
tion: Surgical
Services

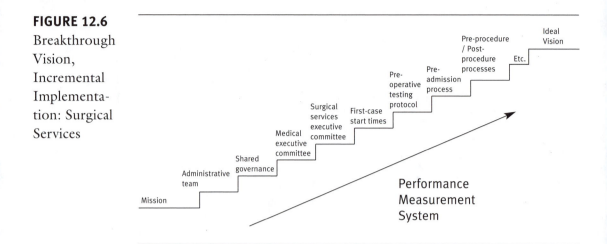

Source: Data from Kelly, D. L., S. L. Pestotnik, M. C. Coons, and J. W. Lelis. 1997. "Reengineering a Surgical Service Line: Focusing on Core Process Improvement." *American Journal of Medical Quality* 12 (2): 120–29.

steps represent specific interventions targeted toward restructuring the governance system to enhance collaboration, partnership, and decision making. Although not explicit in the performance goals, these interventions were essential to carrying out this manager's implicit goals to promote the desired culture needed for future interventions to succeed (see Chapter 8). Subsequent steps represent specific operational improvements that are based on how the multiple goals were defined (Kelly et al. 1997).

The step below the top step is simply labeled "etc." The interventions shown in Figure 12.6 were only the beginning of the ongoing performance improvement culture. Short-term improvement goals, long-term improvement goals, and "just-do" interventions became an integral part of how this service line operated. The unit was also guided by performance gaps identified in the data and those gaps observed by staff and various governance team members (Kelly et al. 1997).

Figure 12.7 illustrates an example of how an improvement team from a medical-surgical unit in a small county hospital (see Chapter 8) documented its performance improvement efforts using the breakthrough vision, incremental implementation framework. Although not as large in scope as the previous example, this 30-bed patient care area found the framework helpful in organizing, documenting, and communicating its efforts. The first step in the lower left corner of the figure documents how the team reevaluated the unit's mission and scope of service and reviewed the unit's history at the beginning of the effort. The step in the upper right corner documents how the team defined its vision in terms of the characteristics of its ideal unit. The team's performance measurement system is represented by the first diagonal arrow beneath the steps. This department already had

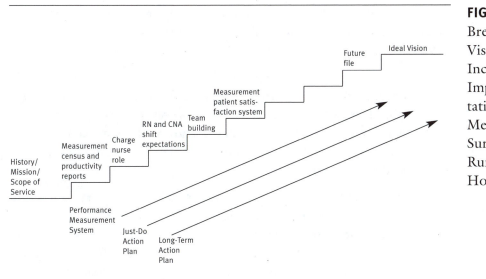

FIGURE 12.7

Breakthrough Vision, Incremental Implementation: Medical-Surgical Unit, Rural County Hospital

a set of clinical indicators in place but lacked financial, productivity, and patient satisfaction measures. The first step represents the first intervention of devising a daily census and productivity report that enabled charge nurses to more effectively allocate and assign staff resources.

When converted to a monthly report, this addition to the clinical performance measures formed the basis of the team's performance measurement system. Recognizing that the patient satisfaction component of its measurement plan would take a bit longer to operationalize, the team worked on other interventions while refining and completing its performance measurement system.

In this case, improvement interventions focused on medium-term goals of clarifying roles and worker expectations and integrating measurement into charge-nurse decision making and staff-meeting agendas. The team also differentiated between short-term interventions—that is, its ongoing "Just-Do Action Plan" (represented by the diagonal line beneath the steps)—and interventions that would take a bit longer to plan and implement, which are represented by the diagonal line labeled "Long-Term Action Plan." Longer-term goals included addressing clinical processes of care and other patient-related improvements. This team used the steps to document the interventions already completed. They used the action plans to track progress of ongoing interventions, and when an intervention was completed, they added a new step to the diagram. The top step is labeled "Future file"; the future file contained creative ideas that the team wanted to remember but was not quite ready or able to pursue at the current time.

The reason this implementation framework is effective in complex systems such as health services organizations is that it is based on the same assumptions of implementing organizational improvements that noted psychologist, Karl Weick, has described in addressing social problems. Weick (1984, 43) defines a small win as

> a concrete, complete, implemented outcome of moderate importance. By itself, one small win may seem unimportant. A series of wins at small but significant tasks, however, reveals a pattern that may attract allies, deter opponents, and lower resistance to subsequent proposals. Small wins are controllable opportunities that produce visible results.

The benefits for managers are that small wins preserve gains and cannot unravel; they require "less coordination to execute"; they are minimally affected by leadership, management, or administrative changes or turnover (Weick 1984, 44). For employees, small wins are less stressful and are easier to comprehend and view as achievable. As a result, employees are more likely to comply with a small-wins intervention (Weick 1984, 44, 45).

Finally, a small-wins strategy acknowledges the dynamic complexity inherent in health services organization, which was discussed in Chapter 4: "Small wins provide information that facilitates learning and adaptation. Small wins are like miniature experiments that test implicit theories about resistance and opportunity and uncover both resources and barriers that were invisible before the situation was stirred up.... [A] series of small wins is also more structurally sound ...because small wins are stable building blocks" (Weick 1984, 44).

Conclusion

Implementing an improvement effort or a more comprehensive performance management system may at first appear intimidating to managers. However, by working backward from an ideal vision, the manager may begin to view the process in more manageable increments. Managers must also realize that implementation is not an isolated event solely for when one is operating from a quality management philosophy but rather an ongoing way of conducting business. The synergistic nature of the strategies of setting goals, understanding purpose, putting into place a performance measurement system, using organizational traction, and implementing improvements and changes according to the framework described in this chapter enhances managers' effectiveness in today's dynamic healthcare environment.

The exercise at the end of this chapter provides the reader with an opportunity to practice identifying mental models that may unintentionally undermine implementation efforts if communicated by management or through change and improvement processes. The exercise also provides a chance to practice identifying unintended consequences. Chapter 13 begins to explore practical team strategies that integrate an understanding of systems thinking.

Companion Readings

Dorner, D. 1996. *The Logic of Failure: Recognizing and Avoiding Error in Complex Situations*, 153–83. Reading, MA: Perseus Books.

Pletcher, M. J., A. Fernandez, T. A. May, J. R. Westphal, C. A. Gamez, D. F. Hersh, and R. Gonzales. 2005. "Unintended Consequences of a Quality Improvement Program Designed to Improve Treatment of Alcohol Withdrawal in Hospitalized Patients." *Joint Commission Journal on Quality and Patient Safety* 31 (3): 148–57.

Werner, R. M., and D. A. Asch. 2005. "The Unintended Consequences of Publicly Reporting Quality Information." *JAMA* 293 (10): 1239–44.

References

Bridges, W. 1991. *Managing Transitions: Making the Most of Change*. Reading, MA: Addison Publishing Company.

Covey, S. R. 1990. *The Seven Habits of Highly Effective People*. New York: Simon and Schuster.

Dorner, D. 1996. *The Logic of Failure: Recognizing and Avoiding Error in Complex Situations*. Reading, MA: Perseus Books.

James, B. C. 2001. "The Scientific Basis of Quality Improvement." Presentation to the 4th International Conference on the Scientific Basis of Healthcare, Sydney, Australia, September 22.

Kelly, D. L., S. L. Pestotnik, M. C. Coons, and J. W. Lelis. 1997. "Reengineering a Surgical Service Line: Focusing on Core Process Improvement." *American Journal of Medical Quality* 12 (2): 120–29.

Kofman, F., and P. Senge. 1993. "Communities of Commitment: The Heart of Learning Organizations." *Organizational Dynamics* 2 (2): 5–23.

Langley, G. J., K. M. Nolan, T. W. Nolan, C. L. Norman, and L. P. Provost. 1996. *The Improvement Guide: A Practical Approach to Enhancing Organizational Performance*. San Francisco: Jossey-Bass.

Nadler, G., and S. Hibino. 1994. *Breakthrough Thinking: The Seven Principles of Creative Problem Solving*. Rocklin, CA: Prima Publishing.

Reason, J. 1990. *Human Error*. Cambridge, UK: Cambridge University Press.

Weick, K. E. 1984. "Small Wins: Redefining the Scale of Social Problems." *American Psychologist* 39 (1): 40–49.

Exercise

Objectives: To practice identifying mental models reflected in selected management approaches, and to practice anticipating unintended consequences.

Instructions

1a. You are a manager faced with initiating an improvement effort. Two contrasting approaches to planning, launching the effort, selecting the team, and defining your role in the effort are shown below. Describe the assumptions or mental models conveyed by the different approaches. Write your responses on a worksheet similar to the one shown below.

Activity	Approach	Assumption(s)/ Mental Model(s) Communicated	Approach	Assumption(s)/ Mental Model(s) Communicated
Planning	Planning by a guidance team composed of management		Integrate planning as part of the team process	
Launching the effort Selecting the team	Change announced by management		Provide information about the problem	
Defining the manager's/ facilitator's role	Team members are appointed by the guidance team or selected by management		Management sets direction and boundaries for participation (e.g., how many, available funds); team members self-selected and/or selected by peers	
	Directs the process; accountable for implementation and results		Manager is coach, trainer, information source, and barrier buster; the entire team and/or system owns accountability for success	

1b. Select your preferred approach to each activity based on the messages that you would like your actions to communicate. You may select an original approach if desired. Describe your rationale for selecting that approach, and write your responses on a worksheet similar to the one below.

Activity	Preferred/Original Approach	Rationale
Planning		
Launching the effort		
Selecting the team		
Defining the manager's/ facilitator's role		

2. Record your responses for this exercise on a worksheet similar to the one on page 218.
    a. Select any process that takes place within a health services organization. Write that process in the center column, column A.
    b. Identify who (person, group, department, stakeholder) influences the process in column B.
    c. Identify who is influenced by the process in column C.
    d. Extend your response one more time. Identify who influences the items in column B. Write your response in column D.
    e. Identify who is influenced by the items in column C. Write your response in column E.
    f. Describe one or two unintended consequences to a change in the process identified in column A.

D	B	A	C	E
Who influences items in Column B	Who influences the process	The process	Who is influenced by the process	Who is influenced by items in Column C

TEAM STRATEGIES

Objectives

- To explore practical team strategies
- To appreciate individuals' differences
- To practice identifying team member strengths

As the department managers at Hospital A sit around the conference table, their minds are elsewhere. One is reviewing financial reports, one is reading mail, one is reviewing his weekly calendar, and one is in and out of the room answering phone calls. The administrator keeps talking, oblivious to the indifference and apathy of the people in the room. Because attendance weighs heavily in the manager's performance appraisal, all managers attend the monthly management team meetings. According to anyone who is asked, the meetings are "a waste of time, but you have to go."

The administrator at Hospital B starts by reviewing the objective of the monthly management team meeting: to provide a forum for information sharing, learning, and collaborative problem solving and improvement. The team consists of the managers within the administrator's scope of responsibility and the human resources, quality, and financial consultants dedicated to her service line. Each participant is leafing through the agenda packet as the administrator reviews the items that will be discussed during the next two hours: "First, each manager will summarize his or her performance indicators for the month. The summary graphs for each department are in your packet, and so is the entire service-line report. Please be sure to point out the positive trends and alert us to potential problems. Second on the agenda is a brief presentation from Manager A about the results of a recent improvement effort and what his team learned from the process. Finally, Manager B will summarize the important points from the conference she attended last week. Does anyone need to add anything to the agenda?" At the conclusion of the meeting, the managers are still milling around the room, asking each other questions, laughing together, and competitively joking about whose performance statistics have shown the most improvement this year.

In both of these examples, highly paid managerial employees are brought together regularly for a meeting. However, the yield from each meeting differs. Predictably, the overall yield from each manager and from the service line as a whole also differ. The collective intelligence of the organization is often an underrecognized variable in the productivity equation, especially when applied to knowledge work like healthcare.

The ability to effectively design and manage teams is an essential management skill. The published literature already offers managers a wealth of information about teams, so this chapter will not review nor summarize them. This chapter will, however, explore some practical team strategies related to the specific concepts described in this book.

Designing Teams

Effective teams do not just happen; they are thoughtfully and purposefully designed. Often the first question asked about a team is, "Who should be on it?" However, the following sequence of questions should be asked any time a manager is considering a team approach on any level, whether on a management team, a project team, a care delivery team, or an improvement team.

1.   What is the purpose of the team (e.g., activity, process, function)?
2.   What is the ideal, step-by-step process or approach to achieve that purpose?
3.   What is the most appropriate structure to support and carry out that process? (Structure includes how people are organized to carry out the process.)

Purpose

When the two meeting examples at the beginning of the chapter are examined according to these three questions, one discovers that the management team meetings in Hospital A do not have a purpose or a defined process. Although its structure is defined, without addressing the first two questions above, this structure has little impact on manager effectiveness and, in turn, on departmental and organizational performance. In Hospital B, the purpose is clearly defined as providing a forum for information sharing, learning, collaborative problem solving, and improvement. The step-by-step process to achieve this purpose is a defined agenda at each meeting that includes discussing performance indicators, sharing successes and individuals' learning, and communicating organizational information from administrators to managers, managers to administrators, and managers to managers. The team members include not only the managers but also a financial officer, a human resources consultant, and a quality department staff member, and the entire team is assigned to the service line. They assist with compiling the performance data, generating management reports, and answering data-related questions at the meetings. Guest speakers are invited to address special topics of discussion. Not only do the managers in this service line demonstrate a high level of individual performance and satisfaction, but overall the service line also consistently demonstrates the highest level of relative improvement year after year, compared to other service lines in the organization.

In redesigning a clinical care team, the following questions should be asked:

- What is the purpose of care in this care setting?
- What is the process of care that will achieve this purpose?
- What is the structure (e.g., types and organization of care providers) needed to carry out this process?

Once the team has been designed, managers must ensure alignment between the team expectations and other components of the organization, particularly leadership and human resources systems, if teams and teamwork are to be successful in the operational setting (see chapters 2 and 5; Kelly and Short 2006).

Process

Aligning Messages

In one project team, the facilitator and manager debrief after the team meeting to clarify their respective responsibilities for the next meeting. The agreed-on guidelines define how the team makes decisions, but when the team members observe the manager and facilitator having a meeting after the meeting, they begin to suspect that the manager has a hidden agenda and is influencing the facilitator toward his agenda rather than the team's agenda. When the unintended messages sent by the post-meeting meeting are realized, the manager clearly explains the assumptions behind his actions. The manager wants to make sure the team has the managerial support necessary to accomplish their goals. Depending on the meeting agenda and resulting discussion, the manager and facilitator often identified issues, information, or follow-up activities that the staff are unaware of because of the nature of their roles. For subsequent team efforts, the manager and facilitator adopt the practice of explaining very early in the project that they need to discuss certain topics without the team. They hope this explanation will proactively prevent any misperceptions associated with "the meeting after the meeting."

Decision Making

Consensus is a widespread approach to decision making in which the team seeks to find a proposal acceptable enough that all members can support it (Scholtes, Joiner, and Streibel 2003). Seeking consensus may, however, reduce decisions to the lowest common denominator (Wheatley 1994). In a team comprising primarily concrete-, practical-, linear-thinking members, how likely is it that an idea posed by the one creative, conceptual team member will gain enough acceptance to be considered a possible solution to a problem? Or conversely, on a team of creative, conceptual innovators who are quickly moving forward on an idea without regard for the practical considerations of implementation, how likely will it be that they embrace the input from the one concrete-, practical-, linear-thinking team member? In either case, the result will be less than optimal. The best result (i.e., improvement intervention) in these two circumstances may come from listening to the "outlier" because that team member's perspective best matches the requirements of the decision at hand. Predictably, the first team shows minimal improvement after its idea is implemented, and the second team is never able to implement its idea.

Using decision criteria is an alternative to consensus. Using criteria does not imply that a team is not accountable for supporting a decision once it is made; it does, however, suggest that decisions will more likely take a diverse perspective into consideration. For example, in one improvement effort, the criteria for pursuing an improvement idea includes the following (Kelly 1998):

- Does it fit within the goal of the effort?
- Does it meet customer requirements?
- Does it meet regulatory requirements?
- Does it remain consistent with the department's/organization's purpose?
- Does it support the vision?
- Does it demonstrate consistency with quality principles?

In this case, team members are expected to question and challenge an idea and, if an idea meets the criteria, the team can pursue it further, confident that the idea is sound. Even though all team members do not completely understand the idea at the time, much time is saved in trying to explain something that is not readily understandable given the individual natures of the team members.

Meeting Schedules and Frequency

Typical meetings are held weekly, biweekly, or monthly, and they generally last one to two hours. Some of the challenges associated with this approach in healthcare organizations include clinical providers not being able to get away from daily patient care duties, team members arriving late because of other competing responsibilities, the need to devote portions of the meeting to updating team members, and dwindling interest as the process drags on.

Consider an alternative approach. If managers use a systematic method for approaching improvements, they will begin to get a sense for the total team time required for an improvement effort. For example, a team may take about 40 hours to complete the various phases of an improvement project. If the improvement effort is constrained by time or dollars, the team is faced with increasing its own productivity or reducing its own cycle time. With this in mind, the 40 hours of time may be distributed in a variety of ways other than one-to-two-hour segments. For example, ten four-hour meetings or five eight-hour meetings may better meet the needs of a particular project. The meetings may occur once a week for ten weeks, twice a week for five weeks, or every day for one week. Based on the particular work environment, a strategy may be selected that balances project-team productivity, daily operational capacity and requirements, the scope of the desired improvement, and project deadlines.

A concentrated team meeting schedule has several advantages:

- It demonstrates the organization's or management's commitment to change.
- It saves duplication and rework associated with bringing everyone up to speed at each meeting.
- It establishes traction by contributing to the elements of creative tension.
- It reduces the cycle time from concept to implementation.
- It forces managers and teams out of the "fire-fighting" mentality into one of purposely fixing not just the symptoms of problems but also the underlying problems themselves.

Structure

For an improvement project team, team composition (how many and who is on the team) as well as meeting frequency and duration should be guided by the purpose and team processes for the improvement effort. The questions that should be asked include the following: "What knowledge is required to design the actual improvement intervention(s)?" "How should the team be designed to support the processes needed to accomplish implementation within the project constraints?"

Focusing on early adopters has been shown to be an effective strategy to get individuals to adopt an innovation. Once approximately 5 to 20 percent of a group have successfully adopted a new process, adoption by the rest of the required group progresses very rapidly (Rogers 1995). According to the Myers-Briggs Type Indicator, approximately 68 percent of the population expresses a personality type that is resistant to change, and 32 percent express a type that is accepting of change (Myers, Kirby, and Myers 1998; Smith 2000). Within the two groups exists an entire continuum of resistance and acceptance. Typically, early adopters of innovations fall into specific Myers-Briggs types.

What does a manager do when faced with implementing improvements when very few early adopters are in the employee pool? This was the case for a manager who needed to obtain rapid buy-in for a large change effort in a department composed mostly of people with resistant personality types. The manager chose a strategy involving a 40-member improvement team, which represented about 25 percent of the total department staff and included formal and informal leaders in the department. Although most of these 40 people fell into the "resistant" group, by involving them earlier rather than later in the process, the manager not only engaged those who readily accepted change but also simultaneously cultivated the critical mass of the resistant types needed to support implementing the improvements. In this way, the speed with which the improvements were adopted and implemented throughout the entire department was greatly enhanced (Kelly 1998).

Team Effectiveness

Although many managers and employees may prefer agreement and harmony, the convergence of diverse perspectives is what supplies the essential elements of creative tension and potentially leads to innovation and improvement, as this quote indicates: "Innovate or fall behind: the competitive imperative for virtually all businesses today is that simple. Achieving it is hard, however, because innovation takes place when different ideas, perceptions, and ways of processing and judging information collide. That, in turn, often requires collaboration among various players who see the world in inherently different ways" (Leonard and Straus 1997, 111).

Although diverse perspectives serve a role in creative tension and foster innovation, they also create fertile ground for accidental adversaries, conflict, and team breakdowns. Managers are challenged to find tools and approaches that enable them to take advantage of differing perspectives while maintaining effective interpersonal relationships within teams and employee groups. How can managers promote friction among ideas while minimizing friction among people?

Talents and Differences

Numerous frameworks are available to help managers understand and appreciate individuals and their differences. Although the taxonomy may vary, each framework defines groups on the basis of common patterns. Studies of large numbers of individuals have resulted in the identification of patterns in their preferences, predispositions, temperaments, learning styles, and strengths. These patterns have been organized and labeled according to various frameworks, including the Myers-Briggs Type Indicator (Myers, Kirby, and Myers 1998), the Keirsey Temperament Sorter (Keirsey 1998), Human Dynamics (Seagal and Horne 1997), and the StrengthsFinder (Buckingham and Clifton 2001). Specific descriptions of these frameworks are not provided in this book, but readers are encouraged to further explore them; see the reference list at the end of the chapter.

When these different frameworks are studied together as a group, patterns may be identified. First, the frameworks recognize that individuals bring differences with them to the workplace. The frameworks identify, categorize, and explain those differences and then provide a concrete and systematic means of recognizing, describing, and understanding them. They also provide a common language and approach for managers and teams within the organization to understand, appreciate, and address differences in the workplace in a positive way. When two of these frameworks—the Myers-Briggs Type Indicator and Human Dynamics—are studied together, some global, cross-cutting dichotomies may also be seen. These include the following dualities: internal and external, practical and creative, data oriented and relationship oriented, concrete and conceptual, linear and lateral, and spontaneous and structured. Although managers may prefer one framework over another, they should begin to look for how these global dichotomies are expressed in themselves, in their employees, and within teams in their organization. Managing the interface of these dichotomies, rather than avoiding or falling victim to them, will enable managers to enhance the effectiveness of both operational working teams and improvement project teams.

Operational Teams

As patient volumes increased, a department grew from five employees to 20 almost overnight. When there were only five employees, the department had functioned like a close-knit family. Yet currently, when new employees came on board, they found themselves thrown into the work with little time to assimilate into the culture and style of the team. For the first time, the department appointed a supervisor to oversee the team, and not long after that the complaints started: "The supervisor never follows through on anything"; "A certain employee is not carrying her load"; or "The supervisor is all talk and no action."

This department had inadvertently set up an accidental adversaries situation between the supervisor and the staff. In Chapter 6, the term "accidental adversaries" is used in relation to double-loop learning and making underlying assumptions explicit. However, accidental adversaries as a result of differences in personalities, styles, and preferences can be a common and unrecognized source of conflict in all kinds of teams.

When the employees in this department took the Myers-Briggs Type Indicator test, the results were illuminating. Eighteen of the 20 department employees were *sensing* types. They preferred the concrete, real, factual, structured, and tangible here-and-now; they became impatient with the abstract and mistrusted intuition. Two of the employees, including the supervisor, were *intuitive* types. They preferred possibilities, theories, invention, and the new; they enjoyed discussions characterized by spontaneous leaps of intuition, and they tended to leave out or neglect details (Myers, Kirby, and Myers 1998). In this department, the supervisor inherently functioned in a manner that was just about opposite to the rest of the department's inherent way of functioning. As a result, misunderstandings, misperceptions, and communication breakdowns became common.

When these differences were understood, the department could put into place specific processes and systems (which were not necessary when there were only a few employees) to minimize the potential breakdowns.

For example, a standing agenda at staff meetings helped the supervisor to stay on task and avoid getting sidetracked. A bulletin board and communication notebook was used to ensure that current and complete information about departmental issues was available to everyone. A performance measurement system was put into place to provide a factual base for evaluating individual productivity and workload.

By understanding and implementing processes designed to meet the differing information and communication needs of the sensing and intuitive types, this department was able to avert further conflict and misunderstanding and focus employees' energy on productive work rather than on perceived supervisory deficiencies.

Project Teams

Just as managers use human resources practices that promote matching an employee's traits with the requirements of the job, managers may also match employees with the various roles and stages required in a change or improvement process. Problems in group processes tend to arise from a mismatch between a process stage and an individual rather than from problems inherent in the individuals themselves. Purposefully engaging individuals at the appropriate time in the process and offering support and requesting patience during other times can enhance the team's and the manager's effectiveness.

A team member favoring a concrete pattern may get frustrated with creating a vision, although he or she will be essential in determining the logistics of the implementation. Someone with an interpersonal or relational pattern can be on the alert for any employee issues related to the changes. An employee with a pattern of seeing the big picture will be invaluable in identifying unintended consequences. A team member who is detail oriented can be an ideal choice for monitoring progress and ensuring follow-through; another member who is action oriented can make sure the team gets moving.

Conclusion

When managers realize that individual mental models and the organizational context surrounding the concepts described in this chapter influence how quality management is operationalized in an organization, they may gain a deeper appreciation for the value of teams as systemic structures. Managers should not only examine their individual mental models as a way to enhance their own personal effectiveness, but they should also incorporate an understanding of this systemic structure while defining the context of the work environment. The manager's responsibility is to select the desired lens through which individuals within the organization and the organization as a whole will view the world. A lens that views differences as complementary talents may result in synergy and success, while a lens that views differences as opposing perspectives may result in conflict, breakdowns, and mediocrity.

Often, team guidelines suggest rules of behavior such as "we will start on time" or "do not interrupt while another person is talking." The exercise at the end of this chapter offers an alternative approach to establishing team guidelines that enhance the team's ability to use team member strengths, increase the team's effectiveness, and improve the quality of the team's output.

Companion Readings

Kelly, D. L., and N. Short. 2006. "Exploring Assumptions About Teams." *Joint Commission Journal on Quality and Patient Safety* 32 (2): 109–112.

Kelly, D. L., M. A. Zito, and D. Weber. 2003. "Using a Stage Model of Behavior Change to Prompt Action in an Immunization Project." *Joint Commission Journal on Quality and Safety* 29 (6): 321–23.

Rubin, I. 1996. "Learning How to Learn: The Key to CQI." *Physician Executive* 22 (10): 22–27.

References

Buckingham, M., and D. O. Clifton. 2001. *Now, Discover Your Strengths.* New York: The Free Press.

Keirsey, D. 1998. *Please Understand Me II: Temperament Character Intelligence.* Del Mar, CA: Prometheus Nemesis Book Company.

Kelly, D. L. 1998. "Reframing Beliefs About Work and Change Processes in Redesigning Laboratory Services." *Joint Commission Journal on Quality Improvement* 24 (9): 154–67.

Kelly, D. L., and N. Short. 2006. "Exploring Assumptions About Teams." *Joint Commission Journal on Quality and Patient Safety* 32 (2): 109–112.

Leonard, D., and S. Straus. 1997. "Putting Your Company's Whole Brain to Work." *Harvard Business Review* 75 (4): 110–19.

Myers, I. B., L. K. Kirby, and K. D. Myers. 1998. *Introduction to Type: A Guide to Understanding Your Results on the Myers-Briggs Type Indicator.* Palo Alto, CA: Consulting Psychologists Press.

Rogers, E. M. 1995. *Diffusion of Innovations.* New York: The Free Press.

Scholtes, P. R., B. L. Joiner, and. B. J. Streibel. 2003. *The Team Handbook, 3rd edition.* Madison, WI: Oriel.

Seagal, S., and D. Horne. 1997. *Human Dynamics: A New Framework for Understanding People and Realizing the Potential in Our Organizations.* Cambridge, MA: Pegasus Communications, Inc.

Smith, R. 2000. *The Seven Levels of Change: The Guide to Innovation in the World's Largest Corporations.* Arlington, TX: The Summit Publishing Group.

Wheatley, M. J. 1994. Self-Organizing Systems: The New Science of Change. Kelner-Rogers and Wheatley, Inc. Conference Proceedings, Deer Valley, Utah, October 17–19.

Exercise

Objective: To practice establishing team guidelines that capitalize on the strengths of team members.

Note

Part I of this exercise may be used to start any group or team discussion. Parts II and III are designed to be used midway through and at the end of a defined team process or project.

Instructions

1. Assign roles in your group. These roles may stay the same or may rotate among team members to provide an opportunity for each team member to practice each role.
   - Select a leader: The leader is responsible for ensuring that the group expectations are completed within the time allotted and that the group does not spend too much time on one item.
   - Select a scribe: The scribe is responsible for recording the highlights of the discussion.
   - Select a timekeeper: The timekeeper will keep the group informed about how much time remains for the meeting or session.

2. Select and agree on group rules: These rules represent guidelines and expectations for how individuals and the group will function to promote the accomplishment of the team's assignment. As a start, the following rules are suggested:
   - Give your full attention.
   - Be respectful of others.
   - Accept responsibility for the team's success.
   Add additional group rules as desired.
   -
   -
   -

3. Identify and discuss each team member's strengths and limitations. Record these characteristics on the following worksheet. Use this worksheet as a reference for your team.

Part I: Team Member Strengths Worksheet

Name	My unique contribution to this project team (e.g., experience, education, perspective, skill, background)	What I am least effective at doing (it is not that I am unwilling to try, it is just not my strength)

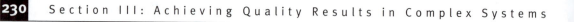

Part II: Midway Team Evaluation and Improvement Plan Worksheet

Scoring Guidelines: 3 = Very effective, 2 = Somewhat effective, 1 = Needs improvement

Item	Score		Improvement Plan
	Individual	Group	
Following team guidelines			
• Giving your full attention			
• Being respectful of others			
• Accepting responsibility for the team's success			
•			
•			
The degree to which team member strengths were contributed			
Name:			
Name:			
Name:			
Name:			
Name:			
The degree to which team member limitations were minimized			
Name:			
Name:			
Name:			
Name:			
Name:			

Part III: Final Team Evaluation Worksheet

Instructions: Review your midway team evaluation and improvement plan. Complete the final team evaluation.

Scoring Guidelines: 3 = Very effective, 2 = Somewhat effective, 1 = Needs improvement

Item	Midway Evaluation Score		Final Evaluation Score	
	Individual	Group	Individual	Group
Following team guidelines				
• Giving your full attention				
• Being respectful of others				
• Accepting responsibility for the team's success				
•				
•				
The degree to which team member strengths were contributed				
Name:				
Name:				
Name:				
Name:				
Name:				
The degree to which team member limitations were minimized				
Name:				
Name:				
Name:				
Name:				
Name:				

EPILOG

The concepts and tools examined in this book come from varied disciplines, yet each has its origins in systems perspective. When used together, their synergy provides managers with a guide to leveraging performance improvement and change efforts. The concept of leverage is derived from physics and is defined as "an advantage for accomplishing a purpose" or an "increased power of action." Leverage is achieved through the action of a lever, which is defined as "a bar used for prying" or "an inducing or compelling force."

In the past, quality management in healthcare has focused on tools to enhance a manager's ability to improve "how things are done" (process) and to "do the right things" (content). In the future, managers will also be required to employ tools that examine underlying thinking and assumptions. This book provides managers with a systems perspective on quality management and with a set of tools that can prepare them for future demands for quality. The tools are intended to address high-leverage, underlying assumptions (i.e., systemic structures) that influence quality management. These assumptions relate to goals, purpose, measurement, traction, implementation, and teams. The figure on the next page illustrates the continuum from low- to high-leverage performance improvement.

A manager must know when to accept and when to challenge underlying assumptions to succeed in an uncertain environment. The ability to understand and fluidly manage the relationship between traditional quality tools and tools that provide a deeper understanding of assumptions and other underlying systemic structures permits managers to continually raise the quality-management lever bar.

When asked how to get to Carnegie Hall, a famous musician replied, "Practice, practice, practice!" The exercises at the end of each chapter provide readers with opportunities to practice the presented concepts and tools. The exercises in the next section offer readers an opportunity to further synthesize these concepts and tools by applying them to a performance improvement effort in a health services organization setting.

FIGURE
Leveraging
Performance
Improvement
in Healthcare

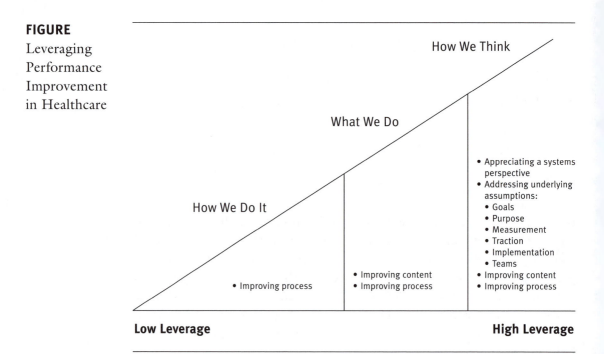

PRACTICE EXERCISES

Practice is crucial to improving. The exercises in this section allow readers to refine their understanding of and familiarity with the theories and processes addressed in the book. The first exercise focuses readers on conducting an organizational assessment to document their organization's current reality. The second exercise involves students in a performance improvement effort in a fictional organization with real-world organizational conflicts. The third exercise allows managers to practice a performance improvement on identified areas of their own organizations using the concepts and tools in this book. These exercises are also available on this book's companion website at ache.org/QualityManagement2.

Exercise 1

Objectives

- To practice using an organizational assessment as a means of documenting current reality and identifying performance gaps
- To practice using the Baldrige National Quality Program (BNQP) Healthcare Criteria for Performance Excellence as a guide for completing an organizational assessment

Notes

1. Students may complete this exercise using the "CapStar Health System Case Study" (see www.baldrige.nist.gov/CapStar.htm). Working managers may complete this exercise using their own organizations as examples.
2. This exercise is adapted from the BNQP Examiner Scorebook (see www.baldrige.nist.gov/06Scorebook.htm) and the 2006 BNQP Healthcare Criteria for Performance Excellence (see www.quality.nist.gov/HealthCare_Criteria.htm).
3. For additional reference, please see Kelly, D. L. 2002. "Using the Baldrige Criteria for Improving Performance in Public Health." Ph.D. dissertation, University of North Carolina at Chapel Hill, School of Public Health. © UMI Company UMI Dissertation Services, Proquest, Ann Arbor, Michigan.

Instructions

1. Select and describe boundaries of the system of interest; the term "organization" will be used to refer to this selected system. You may select a team, a department, a small organization (e.g., an office practice), or an entire organization.

2. Address the following categories within the organization: organizational profile; leadership; strategic planning; focus on patients, other customers, and markets; measurement, analysis, and knowledge management; human resource focus; process management; and organizational performance results. Each of these areas is defined on the Organizational Assessment Worksheet.

3. Read the description of each category (see the Organizational Assessment Worksheet). These descriptions represent the excellence indicators in the BNQP Healthcare Criteria for Performance Excellence. Identify one to three things that your organization does well, according to the excellence indicators. Write those strengths on a worksheet similar to the one provided.

4. Identify and write one to three opportunities for improvement on a worksheet similar to the one provided. The opportunities for improvement represent excellence indicators in the BNQP Healthcare Criteria for Performance Excellence that your organization currently does not address or could improve on. Please note: you are not proposing solutions, but rather identifying performance gaps.

5. Refer to the BNQP Healthcare Criteria for Performance Excellence if you need a more detailed description of organizational activities that represent excellence indicators.

6. Select a priority area for improvement. You may use the Prioritizing Improvement Opportunities Worksheet provided, or you may write your responses on a worksheet similar to it.

Organizational Assessment Worksheet

Organizational Profile

This category is a snapshot of your organization, including the key influences that affect how it operates and the key challenges it faces.

- Briefly describe your organization, including its services; size; geographic community; key patient or customer groups; and current facilities, equipment, and technology as well as the number of patients or clients it serves.
- Briefly describe your organization's key challenges and your organization's current performance improvement system.

This category examines how your organizational leaders guide and sustain your organization. It also examines your organization's governance and how your organization addresses its ethical, legal, and community responsibilities.

Leadership

- Based on the aforementioned indicators, describe one to three key strengths of your organization's leadership.
- Based on the aforementioned indicators, describe one to three areas in which your organization's leadership could improve.

This category examines how your organization develops strategic objectives and action plans. It also examines how your chosen strategic objectives and action plans are deployed and changed, if circumstances require, and how progress is measured.

Strategic Planning

- Based on the aforementioned indicators, describe one to three key strengths of your organization's strategic planning.
- Based on the aforementioned indicators, describe one to three areas of your organization's strategic planning that could be improved.

This category examines how your organization determines requirements, needs, expectations, and preferences of patients, other customers, and markets. It also examines how your organization builds relationships with patients and other customers and determines the key factors that lead to the acquisition, satisfaction, loyalty, and retention of patients and other customers and to the expansion and sustainability of healthcare services.

Focus on Patients, Other Customers, and Markets

- Based on the aforementioned indicators, describe one to three key strengths related to how your organization focuses on patients, other customers, and markets.
- Based on the aforementioned indicators, describe one to three opportunities for improving your organization's focus on patients, customers, and markets.

This category examines how your organization selects, gathers, analyzes, manages, and improves its data, information, and knowledge assets. It also examines how your organization reviews its performance.

Measurement, Analysis, and Knowledge Management

- Based on the aforementioned indicators, describe one to three key strengths of your organization's approaches to measurement, analysis, and knowledge management.
- Based on the aforementioned indicators, describe one to three opportunities for improving your organization's measurement, analysis, and knowledge management systems.

This category examines how your organization's work systems and staff learning and motivation enable all staff to develop and use their full potential in alignment with your organization's overall objectives, strategy, and action plans. It also examines the organization's efforts to build and

Human Resource Focus

maintain a work environment and a staff-support climate that are conducive to performance excellence and to personal and organizational growth.

- Based on the aforementioned indicators, describe one to three key strengths related to how your organization demonstrates staff focus.
- Based on the aforementioned indicators, describe one to three opportunities for improving your organization's staff focus.

Process Management

This category examines key aspects of your organization's process management, including key healthcare, business, and other support processes for creating value for patients, for other customers, and for the organization. This category encompasses all key processes and all departments and work units.

- Based on the aforementioned indicators, describe one to three key strengths of your organization's process management.
- Based on the aforementioned indicators, describe one to three opportunities for improving your organization's process management.

Organizational Performance Results

This category examines your organization's performance and improvement in all key areas: healthcare and service delivery, patient and other customer satisfaction, financial and marketplace performance, human resources outcomes, operational performance, and leadership and social responsibility. This category also examines performance levels relative to those of competitors and other organizations that provide similar healthcare services.

- Describe one to three key areas in which your organization demonstrates strong performance, and describe the nature of the data that document these performance areas.
- Describe one to three areas in which your organization could improve performance, and explain why you selected these performance areas.

Prioritizing Improvement Opportunities Worksheet

1. Review your opportunities for improvement in the first six areas described in the previous worksheet (leadership; strategic planning; focus on patients, other customers, and markets; measurement, analysis, and knowledge management; human resource focus; and, process management).
2. Review the organizational performance results. Select as a priority one of the opportunities for improvement in this area.
3. Explain why you made this selection.
4. List any other opportunities for improvement (listed in question 1) that influence or are influenced by your selected priority for improvement (listed in question 2).
    -
    -
    -

Exercise 2

Objectives

- To provide an opportunity for students to synthesize the concepts in the book by being involved in a performance improvement effort using a case study that presents real conflicts in organizations
- To practice performance improvement in a safe and controlled setting

Notes

1. This exercise is designed for five teams of students. Teams may elect to tackle one of the five performance gaps presented in the case study.
2. The case study that accompanies this exercise is not a business case study (i.e., a detailed description and account of the organization). Rather, it presents enough organizational context for readers to apply the concepts and tools described in this book.

Instructions

1. Read the case study and answer the questions afterward. The questions do not require you to have all the answers, but they lead you to ask the right questions. If you think you need more content information on certain areas (i.e., details about the organization or data), identify that need by defining the questions you would ask to obtain that information.

Case Study

Hospital Background

Last year, the hospital admitted 20,925 inpatients. For 1,000 of these total patient admissions, congestive heart failure (CHF) was documented as the primary or secondary diagnosis. Of these CHF patients, 48 percent were female and 52 percent were male, with a mean age of 63. Approximately 50 percent of these patients had a history of CHF, and approximately 50 percent were newly diagnosed. The average length of stay for a CHF patient with a primary or secondary diagnosis was 4.2 days. The payer mix for the group was 50 percent Medicare, 40 percent private payer, and 10 percent indigent or charity. As part of the hospital's three- to five-year plan to excel in cardiac services, the hospital has decided to focus on CHF as one of its goals this year.

Scenario One: Clinical Performance Gap

Your team represents internists and other clinical staff in an internal medicine practice.

Your interest in improving outcomes in patients with CHF prompted you to join a quality improvement project sponsored by your state quality improvement organization. As part of the project, your team helped clarify guidelines for this patient population in the areas of diagnosis, treatment, and self-management education. Each of the team members has been using these guidelines for the past year.

You have received the evaluation data for the project that show other hospitals' performance in the heart-failure indicators required by the Centers for Medicare and Medicaid Services. The report shows your hospital's overall performance, but you also receive individual reports showing how your CHF patients compare. Your performance is 10 to 20 percent better in each of the indicators compared with the performance of CHF patients in the hospital as a whole.

At the request of the hospital's medical staff president, you give a report on the quality improvement project at the next medical staff meeting. Of the 1,000 CHF patients typically admitted each year, your patients represent only one-tenth, but they demonstrate the best outcomes. As a result, the medical staff president asks your team to lead an effort to improve care to all patients admitted to the hospital with a primary or secondary diagnosis of CHF.

Scenario Two: Operational Performance Gap

Your team collectively represents the manager of the social work department at the hospital.

At the monthly staff meeting, you ask for input on the increasing number of overtime hours that you have observed on the payroll reports. The staff describe their frustrations with how discharge planning is done at the hospital. With the trend toward shorter hospital stays, they are finding that they have more to do in less time. Responsibilities such as arranging transportation, ensuring that follow-up appointments have been scheduled, and arranging home and long-term care are becoming more difficult to accomplish.

Patients who are admitted for CHF and spend a day or two in the intensive care unit pose a particular problem. Many times, the social workers are not notified until the day the patient is supposed to be going home. As a result, everything becomes an emergency, which makes it hard for the social workers to manage their time effectively. You tell your staff that you will initiate an improvement effort on the discharge process and that you will begin with patients with CHF.

Scenario Three: Operational Performance Gap

Your team represents the nursing shift supervisors of the hospital.

A nursing supervisor is assigned to each shift and has the responsibility for clinical and administrative oversight of the nursing staff for that shift. Your specific responsibilities include monitoring and ensuring adequate nursing staff coverage on each shift; serving as a resource to unit charge nurses; assisting with emergencies, such as codes; serving as the administrative liaison for patient complaints that are out of the ordinary or that unit staff are unable to handle; ensuring that admissions, transfers, and discharges of patients between units or departments occur smoothly; and helping to resolve interdepartmental conflicts.

Recently, in an effort to cut costs, the hospital approved a proposal to eliminate the day-shift nursing supervisor. The rationale was that patient care unit managers (some of whom are traditional nurse managers and some of whom are nonclinical administrative managers) are present during the day and should be able to absorb the functions of the shift supervisor. Since this change was implemented, it has become more difficult for you and the other nursing supervisors to do your jobs on the evening and night shifts. One problem is that patients who should have been discharged in the morning are being delayed until the afternoon. Because your bed occupancy is typically around 80 percent, these delays are causing bottlenecks for new admissions from surgery and from the emergency department. In particular, the general medicine floors—including the telemetry unit where the CHF patients are and where approximately 70 percent of the admissions come through the emergency department—are faced with these problems. You have heard the following comments from nurses throughout the hospital:

- "The managers always seem to be at meetings and are never available, so it's like not having a supervisor on day shift."
- "When I take patients downstairs to the lobby to go home, I have always stopped at the outpatient pharmacy to get their prescriptions filled. Lately, I have had to wait in line for 45 minutes!"
- "The doctors won't discharge patients until they see the morning blood work results. Since the lab work isn't drawn until 8:00 a.m., by the time I get the results back and track down the doctor to get the OK for discharge, it's usually close to noon."

Scenario Four: Administrative Performance Gap

Your team collectively represents the administrator for the cardiac service line.

The following departments report to you: the medicine/telemetry unit, the coronary care unit, the thoracic intensive care unit (i.e., heart surgery unit), the cardiac rehabilitation unit, the cardiac catheterization laboratory, and the electrocardiogram and echocardiogram laboratories. You are also the administrative liaison to the cardiologists and thoracic surgeons.

Because the nursing department is decentralized, you have a nursing director who is dedicated to your service line. She has just left your office after describing the complaints she has been receiving from the emergency department: patients are backing up in the emergency department as a result of delays in admitting patients to the general medicine floors, particularly the telemetry unit. The emergency department reports to the administrator responsible for the trauma service line.

You have just been recruited from out of state and are new to this position. You were hired with the expectation that you would improve the coordination of care for patients in your service line. The managers who report to you get together monthly for a managers' meeting. So far you have learned that these meetings have not been very useful in assisting managers with the issues that they consider important. Your predecessor had a traditional command-and-control style, and the managers feel stifled when trying to make the improvements they want to make in their respective departments. You want to help your managers be more effective both individually and as a team.

Scenario Five:
Leadership
Performance
Gap

Your team represents the CEO of the hospital.

You have been in the position for ten years, and your previous position was as a senior administrator. In the past few years, your job has become much more difficult: patients are sicker, lengths of stay are shorter, compliance and other regulations keep accumulating, staff turnover is increasing, and workforce shortages are more prevalent. Every time you go to a professional meeting, you hear of another colleague who has been "reorganized" out of a job. You feel fortunate to have remained in your position for so long, but at its last meeting, the board made it clear that the hospital's quality must improve. Your responsibility is to ensure that the board's requests are carried out. At first this expectation seems unreasonable, given that so many things, such as the nursing shortage, are not under your control. You remember going through a similar crisis in the 1990s, and you thought you had fixed it back then.

Since returning from an executive leadership conference a few weeks ago, you have been doing a lot of soul searching. Your management approach has always worked in the past, but it does not seem to be working anymore. You were intrigued by one of the keynote speakers at the conference, who described the attributes required by healthcare leaders today. The speaker said that "a good leader is one whom others trust and have confidence in following because of that leader's values, vision, capabilities, and expertise in handling unstable and difficult situations"; management of frustration, anxiety, and conflict is particularly admired. Such a leader keeps "human suffering as the uppermost concern" and enables groups to "effectively manage surprises." A truly good leader is "able to identify and help guide innovative projects through various forums—strategic, scientific, economic/business, or political...the type of leader required in healthcare today has detailed knowledge of a variety of disciplines that are required to make a healthcare organization work well and has an insatiable curiosity to learn those disciplines that are unfamiliar" (Peirce 2000, 25–26).

You decide that, starting today, you will reinvent yourself in an effort to meet the board's expectations.

Case Study Questions

1. Select the performance gap that you will improve. In a few sentences, identify the performance gap and the process(es) that comprise this performance area.

2. Describe the customers and their expectations of this process or how you would get them (i.e., voice of the customer).

3. Select one of the systems models (see Chapter 5). Explain where the process(es) described in question 1 fit(s) within the system illustrated by this model.

4. State and critique several possible goal statements for the improvement effort. Use the Goals Worksheet below to organize your thinking. Based on your critique, select the goal you will use for the improvement effort. Refer to Table 8.2 if needed.

Goals Worksheet

Category	Goal Statement or Type of Goal	Pros	Cons

5. Practice the purpose principle by asking yourself the following questions:
   - What am I trying to accomplish?
   - What is the purpose of the process(es) identified in question 1?
   - Have I further expanded the purpose? What is the purpose of my previous response?
   - Have I further expanded the purpose? What is the purpose of my previous response? (Continue expanding the purpose, if needed.)
   - What larger purpose may eliminate the need to achieve this smaller purpose altogether?
   - What is the right purpose for me to be working on? (Describe how this purpose differs or does not differ from the original purpose.)

6. Review the goal from question 4. After completing the purpose questions in question 5, does this still seem to be an appropriate goal? If not, redefine the goal of your improvement effort.

7. Describe a performance measure for this process (i.e., voice of the process) and how the data are collected.

8. Describe the high-level steps of your process using a flowchart.

9. Practice identifying mental models.
   - Identify at least two mental models that may be interfering with achieving a higher level of performance from your process.
   - Describe an alternative mental model for each that could enhance the improvement of your process.

10. Identify and apply any additional continuous quality improvement tools (see Chapter 3) that may help you better understand how to improve your process. Show your work.

11. Describe your ideal vision for this process. Depending on the focus of your improvement, you may do this for the organization or department as a whole and then for an ideal process that is aligned with the overall vision. To help create your vision, you may ask yourself the following questions.

    If your process was the best practice for the community,
    - What would your process contribute to the overall organizational performance and effectiveness?
    - What would patients and families who are receiving care as a result of your process, or who are influenced by your process, say about their experience with your organization?
    - What would employees involved in your process say about the process?
    - What would colleagues around the country who came to learn from your best practice say about your process?

12. Improve your process.
    - Determine if you are solving a problem associated with an existing process or creating a new process.
    - Review your original and/or revised improvement goal(s).
    - Review the purpose of your process.
    - Review your customers' expectations.
    - Review the mental models you selected.
    - Review what you learned from question 10.
    - Define the starting and ending points of your process. Redefine them as needed to support the purpose.
    - Based on the aforementioned information, describe the ideal process that will achieve the purpose you described. Document your process using a high-level flowchart.
    - Check your process against the goal you set for your improvement effort.

13. Review the measure from question 7 that you selected as the voice of the process. Is this measure still appropriate for your ideal process? If not, what would that measure be?

14. Review your goal and your purpose. Would the above measure(s) help you determine if you are working toward your goal and carrying out your purpose?

15. Describe any unintended consequences to any other area, department, process, or entity within or outside of your organization if you improve performance of your process. What measure(s) would help you to be on the alert for them?

16. Describe how the measures from questions 14 and 15 fit into a balanced set of performance measures for the department or organization.

17. For your defined measures, describe the following:
    - Is/are the measure(s) a process, outcome, or structure measure(s)?
    - Where can the data for the measure(s) be found? Who would you contact in the organization to find them?
    - How would you collect the data?
    - How often would you report the data?
    - What would your control charts look like?
    - With whom and how would you share your control charts?
18. You have defined the purpose and described the ideal process. Determine the ideal structure to carry out this process—that is, who and how should the process be carried out to best achieve the purpose?
19. Describe an implementation plan that takes into consideration the concepts described in Chapter 12.

Reference

Peirce, J. C. 2000. "The Paradox of Physicians and Administrators in Healthcare Organizations." *Healthcare Management Review* 25 (1): 7–28.

Exercise 3

Objectives

- To provide an opportunity for managers to synthesize the concepts by being involved in a performance improvement effort using the actual identified needs in their own organizations
- To practice improvement approaches in a safe and controlled setting

Note

Implementing the results of this exercise in your own organization is not required. However, the exercise requires you to think through and document all of the steps in the exercise as if you were actually conducting this effort in your organization.

Instructions

1. Choose a performance gap or area for improvement based on the organizational assessment in Exercise 1. This should be an area for which you have access to performance data. (If actual performance data are not currently available, you need to define a plan of how to obtain them.) This should be an area that is key to your business strategy and within the scope of your defined business unit or responsibilities. Who would you invite to participate in your improvement, and why?
2. Briefly define the performance gap and the process(es) that comprise this performance area.
3. Describe the customers and their expectations of this process or how you would get them (i.e., voice of the customer).

4. Select one of the systems models (see Chapter 5). Explain where the process(es) described in question 2 fit(s) within the system illustrated by this model.

5. State and critique several possible goal statements for the improvement effort. Use the Goals Worksheet below to organize your thinking. Based on your critique, select the goal you will use for the improvement effort. Refer to Table 8.2 if needed.

Goals Worksheet

Category or Type of Goal	Goal Statement	Pros	Cons

6. Practice the purpose principle by asking yourself the following questions:
   - What am I trying to accomplish?
   - What is the purpose of the process(es) identified in question 2?
   - Have I further expanded the purpose? What is the purpose of my previous response?
   - Have I further expanded the purpose? What is the purpose of my previous response? (Continue expanding the purpose, if needed.)
   - What larger purpose may eliminate the need to achieve this smaller purpose altogether?
   - What is the right purpose for me to be working on? (Describe how this purpose differs or does not differ from the original purpose.)

7. Review the goal from question 5. After completing the purpose questions in question 6, does this still seem to be an appropriate goal? If not, redefine the goal of your improvement effort.

8. Describe a performance measure for this process (i.e., voice of the process) and how the data are collected.

9. Describe the high-level steps of your process using a flowchart.

10. Practice identifying mental models.
    - Identify at least two mental models that may be interfering with achieving a higher level of performance from your process.
    - Describe an alternative mental model for each that could enhance the improvement of your process.

11. Practice infusing a different way of thinking into your improvement process.
    - Identify someone in your organization who appears to think in a different way than you do. Using the descriptions in Chapter 12, explain what led you to choose this person.

- Review with this person your progress so far on this exercise.
- Ask for this person's perspective and critique. Describe how this perspective complemented or contradicted your own.
- Describe how you will or will not incorporate this new perspective into your improvement process.

12. Identify and apply any additional continuous quality improvement tools (see Chapter 3) that may help you better understand how to improve your process. Show your work.

13. Describe your ideal vision for this process. Depending on the focus of your improvement, you may do this for the organization or department as a whole and then for an ideal process that is aligned with the overall vision. To help create your vision, you may ask yourself the following questions:

    If your process was the best practice for the community,
    - What would your process contribute to the overall organizational performance/effectiveness?
    - What would patients and families who are receiving care as a result of your process, or who are influenced by your process, say about their experience with your organization?
    - What would employees involved in your process say about the process?
    - What would colleagues around the country who came to learn from your best practice say about your process?

14. Improve your process.
    - Determine if you are solving a problem associated with an existing process or creating a new process.
    - Review your original and/or revised improvement goal(s).
    - Review the purpose of your process.
    - Review your customers' expectations.
    - Review the mental models you selected.
    - Review what you learned from question 12.
    - Define the starting and ending points of your process. Redefine them as needed to support the purpose.
    - On the basis of the aforementioned information, describe the ideal process that will achieve the purpose you described. Document your process using a high-level flowchart.
    - Check your process against the goal you set for your improvement effort.

15. Review the measure from question 8 that you selected as the voice of the process. Is this measure still appropriate for your ideal process? If not, what would that measure be?

16. Review your goal and your purpose. Will the above measure(s) help you determine if you are working toward your goal and carrying out your purpose?

17. Describe any unintended consequences to any other area, department, process, or entity within or outside of your organization if you improve performance of your process. What measure(s) would help you to be on the alert for them?
18. Describe how the measures from questions 16 and 17 fit into a balanced set of performance measures for the department/organization.
19. For your defined measures, describe the following:
    - Is/are the measure(s) a process, outcome, or structure measure(s)?
    - Where can the data for the measure(s) be found? Who would you contact in the organization to find them?
    - How would you collect the data?
    - How often would you report the data?
    - What would your control charts look like?
    - With whom and how you would share your control charts?
19. You have defined the purpose and described the ideal process. Determine the ideal structure to carry out this process—that is, who and how should the process be carried out to best achieve the purpose?
20. Describe an implementation plan that takes into consideration the concepts described in Chapter 12.

JOURNAL EXERCISE

Although reflection plays an important role in personal learning, it is not practiced often in today's demanding work environments. This journal exercise section provides readers with a structured opportunity for reflection on how the concepts discussed and the readings recommended in this book can be applied to circumstances and challenges in the actual work setting.

The three types of questions posed in the Journal Entry Form serve different purposes. First, asking readers to identify key points to remember allows them to personalize their own learning. Depending on a reader's experience and current circumstances, one topic may be particularly relevant to one reader, but the same concept may be repetitive or routine to another reader. This question asks readers what lessons are important to them rather than instructing readers to consider someone else's perspective.

Second, asking readers to list the questions that arise as a result of the readings emphasizes the importance of posing questions. As managers and leaders mature in their roles and fine-tune their critical-thinking skills, they discover that asking the right questions is essential to their effectiveness. Although readers, particularly students, may be accustomed to striving for the correct answers, they should know that journal questions are intended to encourage the practice of formulating good questions.

Finally, asking readers how the concepts offered can be applied to their own career roles, goals, and experiences helps solidify the main focus of this book: to apply quality management.

Following is a Journal Entry Form that may be used for the journal exercise. This form is also available on this book's companion website at ache.org/QualityManagement2.

Journal Entry Form

Name:
Date:
Title of the reading:
Author:
Source:
Number of pages:

1. Key points that I would like to remember from this reading. (Write at least one point, but no more than five.):
    a.
    b.
    c.
    d.
    e.

2. New questions that I have as a result of this reading. (Write at least one question, but no more than three.):
    a.
    b.
    c.

3. Ways I can use the information from this reading or how the information in the reading helps explain a particular situation that I have observed or experienced. (Please be specific. Your answers may be related to your work role, your career goals, or your personal effectiveness.)

INDEX

ABOUT THE AUTHOR

Diane L. Kelly, Dr.P.H., M.B.A., R.N., holds the appointment of assistant professor (clinical) at the University of Utah College of Nursing and adjunct assistant professor at the University of North Carolina at Chapel Hill Public Health Leadership Program. She also holds teaching responsibilities at Weber State University Health Administration Services Program and at Duke University School of Nursing. Dr. Kelly also serves as faculty for continuing professional education programs, including Project HOPE's Health Care Management training program in Central and Eastern Europe.

Dr. Kelly earned a B.S.N. from West Virginia University, an M.B.A. from University of Utah, and a Dr.P.H. in public health leadership/health policy and administration from the University of North Carolina at Chapel Hill. Dr. Kelly's education and 30 years of experience in not-for-profit, academic, and for-profit health services organizations allow her to use a hands-on, patient- and practitioner-friendly teaching style.

Dr. Kelly served as a member of the board of examiners for the Baldrige National Quality Program from 1999 through 2001 and currently serves as an active member of the Editorial Advisory Board for the *Joint Commission Journal on Quality and Patient Safety*. Her efforts have been the subject of peer-reviewed articles and other publications nationwide, including the *Wall Street Journal*.